Healthcare Teamwork

DATE DUE

The Library Store #47-0152

Healthcare Teamwork

Interprofessional Practice and Education

Second Edition

Theresa J.K. Drinka, PhD,
and Phillip G. Clark, ScD

Forewords by
Ron Stock, MD, MA,
and DeWitt C. Baldwin Jr., MD

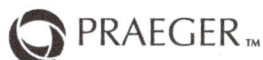 PRAEGER™

An Imprint of ABC-CLIO, LLC
Santa Barbara, California • Denver, Colorado

Library of Congress Cataloging-in-Publication Data

Names: Drinka, Theresa J. K., author. | Clark, Phillip G., author.
Title: Healthcare teamwork : interprofessional practice and education / Theresa J.K. Drinka and Phillip G. Clark ; forewords by Ron Stock and DeWitt C. Baldwin, Jr.
Other titles: Health care teamwork
Description: Second edition. | Santa Barbara, California : Praeger, An Imprint of ABC-CLIO, LLC, [2016] | Preceded by Health care teamwork : interdisciplinary practice and teaching / Theresa J.K. Drinka and Phillip G. Clark ; foreword by DeWitt C. Baldwin, Jr. 2000. | Includes bibliographical references and index.
Identifiers: LCCN 2016015731| ISBN 9781440835094 (print : alk. paper) | ISBN 9781440845369 (pbk. : alk. paper) | ISBN 9781440835100 (eISBN)
Subjects: | MESH: Patient Care Team | Interprofessional Relations
Classification: LCC R729.5.H4 | NLM W 84.8 | DDC 362.1068—dc23
LC record available at https://lccn.loc.gov/2016015731

ISBN: 978-1-4408-3509-4 (hardcover)
ISBN: 978-1-4408-4536-9 (paperback)
EISBN: 978-1-4408-3510-0

20 19 18 17 16   1 2 3 4 5

This book is also available as an eBook.

Praeger
An Imprint of ABC-CLIO, LLC

ABC-CLIO, LLC
130 Cremona Drive, P.O. Box 1911
Santa Barbara, California 93116-1911
www.abc-clio.com

This book is printed on acid-free paper ∞

Manufactured in the United States of America

Contents

Foreword

"Will I do better if my care is delivered by a team? Will my chance of having a better outcome improve? This is what I value. This is the bottom line."
—Jessic Gruman (1953–2014)
Founder and President of Center for Advancing Health[1]

We have embarked on an era in which the question is not whether we incorporate or utilize an interprofessional healthcare team (IHT), but rather how we transform the healthcare system in which the IHT is the standard of care across all sectors of the healthcare system. Since Dr. DeWitt Baldwin's eloquent first edition Foreword (2000), in which he outlined the historical four key points of IHT development over the past century, clearly a fifth moment in history has emerged. Over the past 15 years, the health reform environment has dramatically shaped, or is shaping, the way in which we view both "health" and the manner in which health care is delivered. The emergence of primary care as foundational and the organization of practices into "medical homes," the realization that safe care is not always the standard,[2] the recognition that patient stories and experiences matter, and the unsustainable mounting cost of care have all led to national and state health policy changes resulting in the most comprehensive reform in 50 years.[3] Federal support through the Institute of Medicine, the Agency for Healthcare Research and Quality, and the Center for Medicare and Medicaid Innovation that focuses on care that is accountable and transparent is requiring the healthcare industry to rethink its business model, embracing the "Triple Aim" as the primary measure of quality to improve population health at an affordable cost, while at the same time improving the patient's experience of care.[4]

The lessons learned in the past few years are that our healthcare system is broken and cannot be fixed by doing more, or less, of the same. It is a complex system with a growing number of complex patients with chronic conditions, many health conditions that can be prevented by intervening further "upstream," and an expanding aging population that will stress the current system. The solutions proposed are many, but core is the requirement of a different system of care that relies on a multiprofessional caregiver workforce working together collaboratively with individuals, families, and communities, using an interprofessional team approach.

Building on the theory and core principles developed over a number of decades and expertly conveyed in the first edition, this revision continues to provide a roadmap for practice and healthcare facility staff across the care continuum, but with additional cases and scenarios that expose its relevance in the current healthcare milieu. Appropriately, the addition of a chapter on better understanding the role of the healthcare organization, the "business of medicine," and its relationship to the team brings a valuable broader perspective and opportunities for teams to impact the larger system of care. Additional emphasis on the role of teams in engaging patients to be participants and partners with their healthcare team will assist developing teams in maintaining a "north star" patient-centered approach to achieve positive patient experiences and mutually agreed upon outcomes.[5] Clearly, this will require a workforce that is trained in teamwork, creating the relationships required between professionals, both within the practice and with hospitals and communities, to deliver the team-based care processes providing effective, efficient care that is based on value, not volume.

But teams don't just happen, with most clinicians and healthcare staff ill-prepared to work in a team. Telling professionals from different disciplines to work together and not providing them the training and incentives to be a successful team will not work, and in fact may be harmful to patients and staff alike. This edition emphasizes the important need to match the team behaviors, skills, and ethical considerations required in a practice setting with the educational approaches utilized in our health professional institutions.[6] This will require us to move beyond the segregated classroom and workshop-oriented continuing education approaches into alternative training venues and models, such as community clinical practice "laboratories" that facilitate ongoing peer networking and training paradigms that utilize an interprofessional community-oriented approach within the context of real-life clinical care experiences.

We must also not forget the needs of existing practices and clinical teams that aspire to develop their teamwork and improve team-based care processes. These are the practices that our health professions students will be looking for and expecting to be available to them as they enter the workforce. New continuing education training paradigms will be needed to transform these clinical delivery systems and develop the healthcare practice leaders needed to mentor and sustain this model of care.

Finally, moving toward team-based approaches and promoting IHT development are not without health policy, cultural, and practical challenges/barriers, thus requiring the need to develop a healthcare delivery environment in which IHT approaches are required, or at least encouraged and incentivized to exist. We need licensing boards to acknowledge, broaden, and incentivize roles nonphysician caregivers provide; encourage financial models to sustainably support clinical practices that integrate care and promote collaboration between primary care providers (PCPs) and specialists across care settings; and acknowledge care delivery encounters that occur by multiple providers in the same day, in nontraditional care settings and through such alternative methods as telehealth.

Interprofessional healthcare teams are no longer a "good to have," but they must be the standard of healthcare delivery in all settings. It is imperative for us to develop and nurture this work if we expect to get the quality health outcomes we desire for our children and future generations. Though seemingly an easy concept to endorse, the practical application of IHTs is difficult without the marriage of the knowledge, skills, and experience that is well outlined in this book, and the will and leadership to implement it.

Ron Stock, MD, MA
Associate Professor, Family Medicine
Oregon Health and Sciences University
Portland, Oregon
Director of Clinical Innovation
Transformation Center, Health Policy and Analytics Division
Oregon Health Authority

Foreword to the First Edition

I am tempted to begin by saying that it has taken nearly a century for this book to be written. But such a provocative statement obviously demands an explanation.

As far as we know, the first formal proposals for assembling a team of health-related professionals to provide patient care in this country appeared in the early 1900s, when Richard Cabot, working in the Outpatient Department of the Massachusetts General Hospital, called for the "teamwork of the doctor, the educator, and the social worker."[1] This concept was echoed shortly thereafter by Michael Davis and Andrew Warner at the Boston Dispensary. It is of interest that these physicians all worked in outpatient departments, or what are now called ambulatory care clinics. Also, nurses were specifically not included in these teams. For one thing, at that time, nurses were not considered professionals; and, for another, their skills and contributions were still deemed to be subsumed under those of the physician. Finally, it is noteworthy that the impetus for the call for such teamwork arose not from patient care needs so much as from a professional concern—the threat of increasing specialization in medicine. All three of these physicians believed that the generalist physician was being gradually supplanted or displaced by the emerging specialists in medicine. Adding the social worker and the educator, then, was seen as assisting the specialist to maintain and preserve the broad social and educational perspectives of comprehensive patient care.

Despite this admirable, if hierarchically conceived, notion, the introduction of a concept such as interprofessional or interdisciplinary teamwork, especially for those whom we now refer to as ambulatory or primary care patients, was groundbreaking and significant.

Although the development of specialty-oriented, multidisciplinary, medical, surgical, and mental health teams became commonly accepted in the following decades, it took over half a century for the concept of interdisciplinary healthcare teams to become fully realized, as occurred during the community health center movement of the 1960s. In turn, this led to a major federal initiative to provide training for health professionals assigned to, or aspiring to become members of, the proposed primary care–oriented interdisciplinary healthcare teams. It took still another decade or two for such teams to be seen as essential in the care of a growing and poorly attended geriatric population.

So why did it take the rest of the century to produce this book? Largely, because it has taken that amount of time and experience to begin to separate the varying forms and functions of current and emerging interdisciplinary healthcare teams from their historical antecedents, and to be able to generalize about the specific and essential elements of teaming and teamwork in health care. It also required an important shift from the medical model of the first half century to the health care model of today. Perhaps another way to elaborate on my provocative lead statement would be to look at this book from the standpoint of how persons involved at four key points in the development of interdisciplinary healthcare teams—in 1920, 1950, 1975, and today—would have viewed it.

In 1920, the theory and content of the book would have been virtually unintelligible to the authors of the initial proposals for teamwork. It would probably have been perceived and received with the same sense of incomprehension as were the interstellar rocket exploits of the cartoon strip character Buck Rogers nearly 50 years ago, or the wrist watch telephone of Dick Tracy—both of which have since become a reality. While the ideological values of better patient care would be shared, the pervading power and control of the medical profession and of the hospital clinic setting would have made the discussion of problems such as leadership and conflict appear irrelevant or absurd.

Even in 1950, it is doubtful if Martinsky and George saw their early community-based healthcare teams as much more than an immediate, innovative, practical way to deliver more effective medical care to address specific patient needs. Once again, the detailed discussion of values, leadership, decision making, relationships, power, and conflict elaborated by Theresa Drinka and Phillip Clark in these pages would not have been perceived as important or even relevant for a physician-led team. Even those of us who pioneered the early interdisciplinary educational endeavors of the time with their underlying ideological aims of egalitarianism viewed these efforts as logical and appropriate, but hardly generalizable to the entire spectrum of health professions education. It should also be noted that with the exception of George Szasz at the University of British Columbia, all these efforts occurred at the periphery of major institutional settings.

By 1975, the Community Health Center Movement had made the specific training of professionals for effective teamwork seem essential, but the theoretical models still came largely from the field of group dynamics and were heavily influenced by the ideologies of the time. The need to "prove" that the team concept was successful often precluded any systematic attempt to look more closely at the problems and processes of team care. The only seemingly egalitarian models came from the academically oriented team training programs funded by the government or the emerging use of teams in business. There were some real efforts to summarize and systematize the early experience and learnings of that time, some of which were quite sophisticated and deserve reexamination. Indeed, it is tragic that most of those communications have been essentially "lost" to the participants in the recent renewal of interest in interdisciplinary healthcare teams, partly because there were few, if any, venues for publishing that work and partly because the intent and focus of that phase of development were more on training and not on a broad spectrum of real-life, interdisciplinary healthcare team practice. Another way of putting it would be to say that the emphasis in 1975 was on the "team" as a unique, ideological construct, rather than the more realistic goal of efficient and cost-effective delivery of patient care. The constraints and demands of the environing healthcare systems were largely avoided by a focus on one specific component of care.

Today, as Drinka and Clark make clear, the emphasis has shifted to teams as desirable and appropriate means toward the end of better patient care—a focus on "means" rather than "ends." It fully accepts and deals with the arena of intrateam dynamics, as well as with that of the interface between the team and the dominant healthcare system. Equally important, it clearly distinguishes between interdisciplinary healthcare teams and the fashionable use of working teams in business and industry, while referencing the latter experience. As opposed to the highly structured, "set" teams of the 1970s—formed to meet predetermined and prescribed needs—modern interdisciplinary healthcare teams are more flexible, functional, and based on identifying realistic patient care and health professional needs as well as environing constraints.

Reading this book makes one aware of how far we have come. Indeed, one is reminded of a statement attributed to Anaïs Nin: "We don't see things as they are; we see things as we are." Perhaps, we are finally ready to see teams as they really are. For all of their frustrations and the "roller coaster" history of past and present interest and investment in interdisciplinary healthcare teams over the past 50 years, the current thrust, both on the campus and in practice, seems ready to take off and will be effectively guided by this timely and thorough contribution.

This is the book we have all been waiting for. It is broad, comprehensive, and practical, as well as a conceptual guide to teams and how to "team" with other health professionals in the service of a broader concept of patient care. Perhaps more importantly, the book focuses on the specific contributions to and problems of this process for the health professionals involved. Especially helpful and illuminating are the many tables listing detailed steps and concepts for consideration in team development and maintenance and the extensive use of clinically derived and oriented real-time, and "real-team," illustrations. It should be required reading for anyone who is currently involved, or planning to become involved, with interdisciplinary healthcare teams, as well as for the healthcare administrators who must ultimately understand and support them.

DeWitt C. Baldwin Jr., MD
Scholar-in-Residence
Accreditation Council for Graduate Medical Education
Chicago, Illinois

1

Introduction

We start this introduction by stating our purpose in writing this new edition of our book. It is to continue to provide a foundation for understanding the complexity of interprofessional healthcare team (IHT) practice and education, based on our many years of experience working in interprofessional practice (IPP) and interprofessional education (IPE) settings. Readers who finish this book will have a better understanding of the key knowledge and skills required for IHT members and how educators can best develop and sustain programs to teach these to students and practicing healthcare professionals.

To achieve this outcome, we have kept those sections of the original edition that focused on key aspects of IHT practice, including the development of models of team functioning and development. However, we have also added new chapters in key areas that have emerged over the past 16 years that reflect evolving clinical and educational practice. We believe that our original edition has become an important resource and reference for clinicians and educators alike, and our goal is not to change what we consider the core elements of both IPP and IPE.

We recognize that new care models, methods, and modalities utilizing IHTs are being designed, implemented, and studied. However, our goal is not to get swept up in these new developments, as promising as they might be. By adding new elements and chapters to our original edition, we have avoided evaluating emerging initiatives in clinical or educational practice with IHTs. Rather, we want to stick to "the basics" that have always been the core foundation of IPP and IPE and that will remain the bedrock of IHT practice regardless of the latest trends.

Therefore, we begin this book by pondering the essence of good health care and the role of interprofessional teamwork in that care. The questions of when an IHT is appropriate and what kind of IHT will deliver the most efficient and effective care are difficult but necessary queries in this time of high concern for the cost of health care. It is evident to us that one IHT does not equal another IHT. Also, perceptions of what constitutes a well-functioning IHT are very different among administrators, clinicians, and patients, as exemplified in the following case.

Box 1.1   The Case of Ruth Saxon

I was engaged by a university to conduct a workshop on healthcare teamwork. As part of my itinerary I was scheduled to visit a healthcare facility used by several universities for student training. The facility administrator was very proud of one of his teams and wanted me to see how well it functioned, so he invited me to attend the team's care-planning meeting. I joined the meeting just as it began.

The RN (at the head of the table) was presenting the problems of the resident, Ruth, who was seated to the nurse's right with her husband, George. An activity therapy assistant, a social worker (recently graduated with a BSW), and a dietary assistant (who was head of the dietary department) were also at the table. The nurse stated that the purpose of the meeting was to review the interprofessional care plan for Ruth. It was evident Ruth had suffered a stroke and had expressive aphasia with involvement on her right side. She kept feeling her right hand and wincing as though it hurt. The RN was the first to present, saying that Ruth seemed to be doing well on her medications: Coumadin, hydrochlorothiazide, alendronate, Lanoxin, and Benadryl. The RN mentioned that Ruth's occasional urinary incontinence was under control. When Ruth looked startled to hear about her complex medication regimen, George held her hand. George said that his main concern was refinancing their house so he could pay the medical bills. George said he was trying to consolidate his bills and needed Ruth's signature to get a loan to pay his bills so that he would only have one monthly payment. He kept repeating, "if only she could sign her name, I could get squared away and wouldn't have to worry about losing the house." Team members nodded their heads in empathy, but no one spoke.

The activity therapy assistant spoke about Ruth's need to attend more social activities, because she wasn't meeting her goal of five per week. George said he visited Ruth every day and asked if that counted. The therapy assistant simply repeated that Ruth should attend more group activities.

The dietary technician reported Ruth wasn't drinking enough water but said she had addressed Ruth's eating problems by giving her large-handled implements. George said he offered Ruth fluids when he was there and wondered how he could get her to drink more water. The dietary technician said she didn't care how he did it but that Ruth needed more water.

The social worker reported that Ruth received and read her own mail. She said that George visited Ruth twice a day and they appeared to have a strong relationship.

At this point, all team members had given their reports. The nurse declared the care-planning meeting was over. She turned to Ruth, offered her a pen, and asked her to please sign the care plan.

What I witnessed was efficiency *without* effectiveness. The goal of this team was the team's process rather than good patient care. This case is a metaphor for inept teamwork. It is an example of how the completion of care tasks by multiple providers is only useful if those tasks address the patient's perceived needs and do so as part of an integrated and thorough care plan. What was perhaps most bothersome about this experience was the facility administrator's lack of understanding of what comprised an effective care-planning meeting. It was apparent he equated good teamwork with meeting the paperwork requirements of regulators.

The Accelerating Complexity of Interprofessional Teamwork

This book is about the practice and educational implications of effective and efficient interprofessional teamwork in health care. As such, it discusses a topic that has both an interesting and a distinctive history and increasing relevance. As we published the first edition of this book in 2000, forces of change were sweeping through the U.S. healthcare system. Rapid change continues to accelerate as this second edition goes to press in 2016. We present this book with great humility, since health care is changing faster than any book can realistically capture. In 2010 the Affordable Care Act (ACA) was passed in the United States. The underlying mandate of passage was that the bill had to be fiscally responsible and not increase the federal deficit. As a result of the passage of the ACA, U.S. health care is purporting to create systems of care delivery that provide the best care to the most people at the least cost.

In the shadow of massive change in health care, we reflect on what we wrote in the first edition: "We find that in some ways health care has not changed much in the last 100 years. In the year 2000, as in 1900, a new era of technology is emerging; a tension exists in health care between those who think that therapies should be research- and data-driven and those who offer cures with herbal and other alternative remedies; and non-physician health care providers are struggling to re-define themselves, resulting in independent channels of education and practice." These statements remain true in 2016.

Despite the similarities, the healthcare picture in 2016 is increasingly more complex than it was in 2000. New technologies using genetic testing to modify treatment for specific patients, breakthroughs in immunotherapy, and the development of designer drugs promise to conquer diseases and provide longer lives for people who develop previously deadly diseases. Aided by the computerization of healthcare records, by informatics, the Internet, and also by apps for health tracking devices, sophisticated data tracking and implementation systems have burgeoned in the past 16 years. These systems allow patients to better track their health care and have allowed healthcare systems to track patient data and use that data to give feedback to healthcare professionals on their performance and efficiency.

Although health system responses to patients' perceived needs are rapidly changing, it is doubtful the actual needs of patients have changed much in 16 years. Despite their level of vigilance, patients still need to trust their providers to provide the best care possible for their conditions. The major difference is that many patients are more educated and more sophisticated about health care than they were in 2000. As patients become more involved in their health care, they may become less trusting of the physician, nurse practitioner, or physician's assistant as ultimate authority in their care. At the same time, physicians and other providers are often caught between the patient's needs and the determinations of health insurance providers to deny recommended care.

Thanks in large part to the Internet, in 2016 more patients want to play an integral role in setting the course for their health care. Patients increasingly attempt to do their own medical research before seeking medical care and some patients prefer pseudoscience to real science.

Patients might obtain their healthcare information regarding medications and prosthetic devices from the Internet and television commercials. The Internet is replete with *experts* alerting the public to remedies they never knew they needed and touting the benefits of internal body cleanses, diets that eliminate food groups, and prosthetic devices that needlessly cause more dependence and atrophy. The information patients receive may or may not be derived through any rigorous scientific methodology. Some patients also have developed less trust in traditional medicine and science, as evidenced by their fear of tested therapies like vaccines.[1]

Patients' ideas about health care don't always match those of the healthcare team. Some patients feel more hopeful or at least more powerful when they can seek out their own relief. While health care has recognized and embraced some alternative remedies like meditation, yoga, acupuncture, and probiotics, it remains skeptical of remedies that have not been vigorously tested. When they finally visit their healthcare provider(s), patients expect to be more involved in their care. However, without coaching, patients are unsure of their position with respect to the healthcare team and what the nature of their involvement should be. If we are to reach patients, we must be more willing to listen and understand the patient's preferred approach to health care.

Health care is beginning to recognize that mental health and physical health are interwoven. Unfortunately, funding structures do not fully support this concept. Consequently, services for prevention and long-term treatment of mental health conditions are inconsistently incorporated into a patient's general medical plan of care. The existence of a mental health issue and/or frailty either in the patient or in the patient's support system can drastically change a patient's prognosis. However, the general healthcare system is not yet well structured to deal with this reality, preferring to focus on more quantifiable physical symptoms and disorders.

Administrators and funding sources for health care tend to focus on disciplines like nursing and medicine and might not recognize the value of other disciplines like social work and psychology. Underfunding certain disciplines makes it more difficult to get an appointment with those disciplines. Subsequently, the disciplines more freely reimbursed might take on problems that keep them from tasks they are more highly trained to perform.

In the following story, the nurse practitioner (NP) expresses the realization that she cannot efficiently address all of the needs of her clinic's most complex patients.

Chris: "For ten years we have been begging management for a social worker to be part of our clinic team. As a[n] NP in a primary care clinic, I realize it only takes one patient who has a myriad of physical needs coupled with an acute mental health problem to throw the entire clinic flow out of whack. There are many days when most of my time is spent dealing with mental health issues that are very time consuming. Medicare and Medicaid only allow referrals to one mental health provider. Patients can get an intake appointment but they wait 10 months for a follow-up appointment. It requires a vast knowledge of mental disorders, community resources, and how those resources actually work to meet the needs of these complex patients. With funding cuts to the community support services, an awareness of the existence of a service is not enough. You have to know what service would most benefit the patient, the capabilities of each service, which services are accepting new patients, and whether the service is still operational."

When healthcare professionals, particularly those in primary care, don't have the resources to meet the needs of patients with complex problems, they might choose to ignore the patients' problems that require a particular skill set or try to adopt new skills to meet the demands of their patients. Some professions, after realizing their deficits and the deficits in the system, have tried to increase the scope of their training programs thinking they can do it all. However, given the increased pace of health care, this approach can dilute their valuable time and might not produce the intended effects.

The Need for More Effective Interpersonal Communications between Providers

The complexities inherent in health care highlight the increasing importance of interpersonal communications between multiple providers, providers and administrators, and providers and patients to achieve effective diagnosis and management. Harmful health care often happens as a result of no communication or a breakdown in communication between several providers who may or may not be from different disciplines, or between providers and patients who may be from different cultures or backgrounds. Learning essential communication skills involves a mix of art and science. Even when healthcare systems hire technically competent providers, the critical thinking, interactional, and team skills might not be adequate to effectively meet the needs of patients.

In the past, the healthcare system has heavily weighted its efforts toward treating acute disorders. Baby boomers are retiring in record numbers and economies of scale are now forcing the political and healthcare systems to address the chronic care needs and costs of this burgeoning population. As the healthcare collective looks at the central issues of decreasing costs and increasing efficiency, it is reconsidering the potential value of teamwork to address complex and intersecting problems inherent in chronic care.

In our collective 70 years of working with healthcare teams as care providers, educators, researchers, and administrators, we have seen many fads come and go. We cannot know if the way the healthcare collective chooses to practice and fund teamwork this time around will stand the test of better health care at lower cost. We can only say that we have experienced functional and dysfunctional teams, as well as interprofessional educational programs that come and go. In this edition of the book we use our knowledge to share what has and has not worked in healthcare teamwork practice and education.

Some Historical Reflections on Interprofessional Teamwork

The delivery of health care has dramatically changed over the past 60 years. The practice of healthcare teamwork has come and gone and returned many times in different forms, subject to the whims of administrators who, when faced with the need to cut the budget, made healthcare teams their first target. We have seen repeated attempts to reinvent the teamwork we practiced and taught in the 1960s, 1970s, 1980s, 1990s, and 2000s. Sometimes these attempts have advanced the practice of teamwork, and other times they have stifled its mature development. We have also seen failed attempts at using technology to improve teamwork.

We recall placing computers in patients' homes in the late 1970s with the intent of improving the home care team's ability to monitor care. This noble attempt resulted in blowing out the electrical circuits in the patients' homes. Although the idea was stellar, it did not match the time and available technology. Since that time, technical aspects of teamwork have advanced to where they can now be used for the benefit of patient and team. An example of this is using online video to collocate disparate teams and provide better health care for rural populations. However, technology does not promote teamwork when practitioners are given aging equipment that is subject to frequent malfunctions. It is also a problem when the programs written for one system are incompatible with those of a provider in another healthcare system.

In the 1960s and 1970s there were Health Manpower grants that promoted healthcare teamwork and education. In the 1970s and 1980s the

Department of Veterans Affairs funded both Health Manpower grants and Interprofessional Team Training Programs that were integrated with educational endeavors for physicians and allied health students. In the 1980s and 1990s the Robert Wood Johnson and Hartford Foundations funded efforts in interprofessional team development and education. However, when economies faltered, many of these programs either contracted or disappeared. Sometimes teams were continued, but without support for someone who could manage the teams' evolution and survival, they did not achieve their intended goals.

Increasingly we are recognizing that the way we fund health care contributes to outcomes.[2] The Institute for Healthcare Improvement (IHI) has initiated its Triple Aim of improving the patient experience of care, improving health populations, and decreasing the per capita cost of health care.[3] The Agency for Healthcare Research and Quality (AHRQ) has initiated a national effort to train healthcare providers to work as teams by developing and promoting their TeamSTEPPS Curriculum.[4] Governmental agencies have funded experiments in healthcare provision.[5] And other funders such as the Josiah Macy Jr. Foundation[6] have gained interest in interprofessional teamwork as a core value of health care. We hope these most recent ventures create permanent positive changes in the way health care is delivered to patients with complex problems. We hope these and other efforts improve the patient experience and address improvements in the general health of populations. Through these efforts, perhaps we can reduce the cost of health care.

A New Vision of Health Care and Healthcare Education

To accomplish the goal of efficient and effective patient care, a new vision of *team* must come from the heart of health care, not just from the educators, clinicians, or administrators. In the past, a major hurdle to mature IHTs has been an inability to build interprofessional team development and maintenance into the fabric of health care supported by continuing educational programs for healthcare professionals. Health and education systems evolve. Funding comes and goes. CEOs change and teamwork's value to the organization changes with them. Forward thinkers have been promoting interprofessional teamwork for more than 60 years. However, teamwork education has followed the money, and when the money is scarce teamwork education fades into the woodwork.

It is no longer acceptable to promote interprofessional teamwork in an institution and leave the execution of it to chance. It is insufficient to promote initial team development training and then leave the team with no extra resources to deliver care as an integrated system. It is equally important to help a team develop and recognize that sophisticated team systems need to be maintained and that team members must be assisted in finding and scheduling time to manage their team structures and processes.

Increasingly, we understand that massive change from the culture of medicine over the past 100 years requires a complete revamping of medical training and clinical education into a model that integrates the disciplines and moves them toward a culture of interdependent learning.[7] If health care is going to evolve in a meaningful way, it needs to continually reexamine its delivery structures but also the structures that educate its workforce. Instead of giving lip service to IHTs, we must examine what they are and what they are not, and why they are not achieving what they need to achieve.

We must be realistic about the effort and resources that are needed to make them work for the patient, while also controlling costs. Healthcare professionals, educators, and administrators, along with their funding bodies and even patients, share responsibilities in making health care work. We believe more than ever that well-planned IHTs are necessary. However, realistic primary and continuing educational programs for interprofessional learning and care must be part of the equation. Their funding cannot be transitory and must become foundational and welded into the entire system of healthcare education.

Difficulties in Interprofessional Training

Comprehensive in-depth training in interprofessional teamwork is the first major hurdle to achieving well-developed and effective IHTs. We recall a difficult effort by an interprofessional group of clinical faculty in the 1970s to develop a teamwork course consisting of a series of didactic lectures and case studies, offered to nine healthcare disciplines, including medicine, nursing, social work, pharmacy, dietetics, occupational therapy, physical therapy, speech pathology, and audiology trainees. Offering the course required approval from the deans of each of the schools. We managed approval from four schools to run the course for a year. However, due to difficulty matching schedules, the course was discontinued. Success required more money than we had to contribute to departments and more influence than any one faculty member had. In most academic settings these issues are still unresolved.

We substituted team practicums, where clinical faculty members from one or several of our active clinical teams supervised students from their discipline. Each student taking the clinical was required to attend a series of lectures and discussions on interprofessional teamwork. A stumbling block to standardizing teamwork learning was the differing lengths of time students were assigned to their practicums. Times ranged from several weeks for undergraduate physical and occupational therapy students, to three months for nurse practitioner students, to nine months for social work master's degree students, to a year for medical fellows.

Another problem for the curriculum was the level of students. The levels ranged from undergraduates to doctoral level. No matter the length of time or level of students, each experience was accompanied with observations and interactions with developed IHTs. While these experiences were all valuable, they led to differing levels of understanding about teamwork.

A second hurdle to well-developed and effective IHTs is establishing teamwork maintenance as secondary to direct patient care. There has been a stubborn unwillingness on the part of administrators to recognize the benefit of highly skilled team managers who have dedicated time for that function. Effective team managers are highly trained in both clinical practice and interprofessional teamwork. Historically, teams gave little credence to managers who did not have clinical credentials, and the notion that team managers had little value if they didn't also see patients was widespread. Some of the problems were with the organization, as team members were squeezed to do more with less. A team manager with no clinical credentials was viewed as extraneous. And a team manager with clinical credentials was pushed to do more clinical work, ultimately forcing that individual to do less team development and maintenance.

A third hurdle to well-developed and effective IHTs has been a lack of time, money, or expectation supporting more highly skilled providers to interact with and teach the lesser-skilled providers, especially across disciplines. There is only limited time to review the results of care. The development and maintenance of IHTs may be our best solution to fragmented, mistake-ridden health care. However, this cannot be your 1980s version of "everyone (including the janitor) sitting around a table" team. This is not your administrator's 2000 "business school measuring short-term costs vision" of team. Nor is it the health providers "stick together with your own kind and when your treatment doesn't work, pass it on to the next discipline" vision of team. It is an interprofessional team that is a lean, efficient, and sophisticated entity for comprehensive healthcare delivery.

Our Approach to the Second Edition of This Book

The first edition of this book focused primarily on the inner workings of the IHT and on teaching the skills needed by care providers enabling them to function on an IHT. This edition additionally focuses on the corporatization of health care and patient participation both in their care and in their interactions with the team. We also focus on the responsibilities of educators and administrators to understand how teamwork education and team structures and functions affect the development of teams and the patients for whom they care.

As hard-core believers in interprofessional teamwork and education, this book reflects our knowledge, biases, and collective wisdom about the requirements for effective healthcare teamwork practice and education, and the impediments to making it all work. We begin by clarifying our preferences for what to call the team, what to call the recipients of care and their relationship to the team, and the use of models.

What to Call the Team

Although we used the term *interdisciplinary* in the first edition, in the interest of reducing confusion, we have switched to using the term *interprofessional* in this edition. With the integration of healthcare technicians and other support staff, it is important to remember that some members of a team might not have a professional code of conduct or requirements for training in ethics. So, in many ways, interdisciplinary is a more accurate term in that it is more inclusive, encompassing team members who are not technically healthcare professionals. However, the convention has evolved to using the term interprofessional, and we will bow to that norm.

What to Call the Recipients of Care

With the advent of the consumer movement and healthcare maintenance organizations, terminology has developed intending to establish a person's involvement in their care (e.g., customer, consumer, client, participant, and partner to name a few). We continue to use the term "patient" over some of the more business-oriented terms, because historically it designates the primary focus for a healthcare intervention as someone with healthcare knowledge helping someone who is ill. While the idea of healthcare consumers sounds good in a business model, in reality, patients are often unable to consciously weigh their healthcare options and choose the best or least expensive model or provider. Patients come to health care because they need help. Healthcare professionals have knowledge beyond what patients have, and effective help requires an element of trust between them.

Patients as Team Participants

We firmly believe that patients, to the extent possible, must be involved in determining their course of health care. In this edition we focus more on the patient and the patient's relationship to the team. While we believe that patients should be actively involved in their care, we question the term "patient-centered care." It reminds us of intimidating pictures portraying a group of healthcare providers in a circle looking down on a helpless bedridden patient. We therefore include a chapter in this edition titled "The Patient as Teacher and Learner" (Chapter 8). In it we discuss, *patient involved care*, a phrase that better describes a patient's interaction with the IHT.

Patients should participate in their care according to their abilities and desires. The responsibility of the patient and/or their advocate to express the patient's needs and desires is not only difficult but also demanding when the patient and/or advocate does not feel up to participating, is mentally compromised, or is emotionally labile. Determining a patient's true mental, emotional, and physical capacity and desire for participation can be very difficult and is one of the responsibilities of highly skilled team members. We believe the patient's needs are central to the team's focus and a patient or designee must be an active participant in the team's work. However, it may be disingenuous to consider the patient a member of an IHT that needs to work on its tasks and processes for healthcare delivery. An important role for the team is to educate the patient in how best to work with the team for better care.

The Use of Models

There are many models of teamwork. It is our belief that you cannot create a mature IHT without a solid plan. The models we provide are based on our experience with IHTs that have succeeded and those that have failed. The models relate to the path of IHTs from inception to maturity. In developing a mature IHT, there are no shortcuts and the ultimate product is relational to the applied effort and available resources. As health care has evolved, many different types of teams have emerged. However, the basic principles of creating long-term and viable IHTs have not changed much since this book was first published. It is our intention that these models provide fuel for dialogue and debate, and they should evolve as our knowledge of IHTs continues to evolve.

The Interprofessional Team Approach to Health Care

There are those who equate teams with groups, and those who recognize teams but do not distinguish between different types of teams. Group development theory is often applied to all small groups. This has contributed in the past to scarcity of funding for research on the development and function of different kinds of teams and groups. If we reduce all teams to groups, and all groups are thought to be the same, then there is no point in comparing different kinds of groups or teams.

This book is based on our experience that groups may be a part of but are not the same as teams, that healthcare teams are different from other kinds of business teams, and that there are different kinds of healthcare teams. The healthcare teams that we write about in this book are IHTs.

Neither every type of patient nor every situation calls for a team approach. Well-developed and efficient IHTs are those that can quickly evaluate a complex situation, define the problems, and determine the most efficient and effective strategies for providing care. Team members participate only when and how they are needed. This type of team requires more initial effort and pays off in the long term. It pays off if the system is stable enough to allow teams to develop around a core element of trust. It is only through mutual trust that errors will be noted as problems to be solved and processes to be improved.

Currently, health care in the United States has a heavy focus on the economic bottom line. Historically, this focus has been one of the controlling forces that prevents teams from treating the patient holistically. However, concern for the monetary bottom line does not account for all problems that make the current healthcare system seem lacking to some and untenable to those who have been hurt or short changed by it. The value systems of all of the players in health care also play a role in the kind of care that is provided and how all participants perceive that care.

In the past we expected doctors to be *know-all gods*. Some providers and some patients might still have that untenable expectation in an environment where knowledge is exploding and the time allowed with patients is imploding. Different healthcare professions differ in their values relative to how health care should be provided. Management professions emerge from a mind-set that differs from healthcare professions, and yet these entities are expected to behave as though they comprise one system with spoken values of efficient, effective, and safe care. Their unspoken values are not as clear, and yet those unspoken values still drive much of health care. Patients often have very strong values related to their care and that of their loved ones, yet patient values can get lost in the shuffle. We ask the readers to reflect on these issues as they are entwined in the creation of IHTs that work both for patients and for the bottom line. We desperately need innovation in health care and must pay close attention to the results of ongoing studies on these issues. Only by team members achieving collaboration with one another and with administrators will innovation happen. We must continue to include administrators and funders in efforts to create and nurture teams that can truly innovate.

We now consider health care a business. Business literature is full of messages about the *learning organization*. In learning organizations, employees at all levels not only learn continuously, but they actively seek new ways to apply their knowledge to help the company and themselves reach and exceed their goals. Similar to differences in values, the spoken goals of health care might not match healthcare's unspoken goals. We must ensure that funders, administrators, providers, patients, and educators elaborate and share their goals for comprehensive health care.

In our interviews with healthcare professionals and patients we have heard about healthcare organizations cutting back on patient care meetings for teams, eliminating meetings for team development, decreasing the standards for hiring certain professionals, and reducing opportunities for healthcare providers to collaborate. These messages are inconsistent with the current rhetoric on integrating teamwork into healthcare systems. So what is the real message of teamwork? We begin this book by placing this question on the table as stimulus for open dialogue among healthcare providers, educators, administrators, funders, and patients. We provide additional cases, exercises, and materials for collective questioning and discussion at the end of this book.

The vignettes in this book are based on interviews with healthcare professionals, administrators, and people who have been patients in a variety of healthcare systems. Details have been changed in the stories to disguise the interviewees and the institutions. We were struck by the caring and concern our interviewees had regarding the state of health care and also with their desire to make it better.

Questions for Discussion

1. What are some *spoken* values your profession espouses about health care and IHTs?
2. What are some *unspoken* values your profession espouses about health care and IHTs?
3. What changes in curriculum could your discipline make at all levels of training to facilitate interprofessional team based care?

Health Care and Teamwork in a Business-Driven Environment

In 2000, when this book was first published, seeds of change had been sown in U.S. health care and were beginning to germinate. The fact that health care had become a sophisticated money-making business became a perfect counterpoint for the efforts of governmental agencies to curb the spiraling costs of health care. Attempts at cost control were focused on quality improvement projects with an emphasis on patient safety. The ultimate goal was efficiency and cost savings. Increasingly sophisticated record keeping and tracking systems allowed healthcare systems, insurers, and governmental agencies to monitor diagnoses and treatments that were easy to quantify.

Healthcare teamwork in 2000 was directed toward teams that managed easily identifiable problems with quantifiable outcomes. In the ensuing 16 years, specialty clinics and surgical teams have improved their records for efficiency, accuracy, and safety. However, similar increases in efficiency were not always replicated in the primary care sector, particularly in patients with multiple interacting chronic problems. Creators of the Affordable Care Act (ACA) in the United States predicted increasing numbers of primary care patients and a decreasing supply of primary care physicians. The impending financial impact of those inevitabilities redirected attention to interprofessional healthcare teams (IHTs) as a way to address the need for efficient primary care. This chapter will explore the realities of IHTs in a business-driven environment.

Escalating Costs and the Corporatization of Health Care

The drive to halt the escalation of healthcare costs over the past 36 years has solidified the corporatization of health care in the United States. Since models for the diverse fields of business and health care were so different, there was a need for common meanings and catchphrases that would come to be used by both management and healthcare professionals. The quality movement that was adopted by business in the 1980s filled that need. Healthcare professionals understood the need for quality and safety, and the goal of healthcare management was to link quality and safety to efficiency and cost effectiveness as it had been done in the manufacturing sector.

Business strategies, models, and philosophy have seeped into health care over the past 36 years, and currently permeate most healthcare models to the point that practitioners might not question the effects of corporatization on their work. Yale University had begun developing the diagnosis-related groupings (DRGs) in the 1970s. By the 1980s, the federal government was looking at a way to contain costs for Medicare and Medicaid and settled on the DRGs as a way to accomplish that objective. In 1983, the U.S. Centers for Medicare and Medicaid mandated the use of DRGs in hospitals as a way to classify hospitalized patients and reimburse hospitals on the basis of case mix.[1] Reimbursement was established by a formula that looked at groupings of patients with specific disorders and the resources needed to treat them. By 1987, the DRGs were in widespread use in hospitals throughout the country.

Healthcare providers not only accepted the new DRG guidelines, they often overinterpreted them as hard and fast rules, thinking they had to discharge patients within the marginal guidelines set. In the early years of their use, DRGs did not include many guidelines on severity of illness, treatment difficulty, or intensity of resources needed to discharge. However, over time, these qualifiers were included in updates to the DRGs. The following vignette illustrates the initial impact of the DRGs:

> **Joseph:** "As a hospital social worker in 1987, I was astounded by how quickly healthcare professionals accepted the DRGs without question. Initially, there was a great push to discharge patients within the recommended guidelines set by the DRGs. If five days were allowed, then the patient had better be ready for discharge by the end of day 5. I recall pleading with physicians who ordered me to find a place for patients who were clearly not ready for discharge or whose home support system had collapsed at the last minute."

In the first edition of our book, we presented the Westside Clinic. We now present the clinic in 2000 and how it might look in 2016.

The Westside Clinic in 2000

By 2000, the DRGs were an accepted part of health care and corporate health care was looking at further ways to save money. In 2000, the Westside Clinic struggled to justify its team approach to care. The clinic operated with an IHT consisting of a registered nurse (RN) with two years of training, a family practice physician, a nurse practitioner (NP), and a social worker with a master's degree (MSW). Like most primary care clinics, its patients were a mix of relatively healthy individuals and the chronically ill. Patients' problems were often coupled with a history of low, unstable income and pressing family responsibilities. Some of the families were struggling with serious mental health or substance abuse issues. Many of the patients, like Mrs. Adams, had physical problems that periodically were accompanied by grief, anxiety, or depression. Mrs. Adams was the caregiver for her husband who, at the age of 52, had recently been diagnosed with Alzheimer's disease. Mrs. Adams also cared for her three-year-old grandson while her daughter searched for work.

Mrs. Adams had adult onset diabetes and rheumatoid arthritis. She had recently been treated for an episode of major depression. Through close collaboration, the clinic team managed Mrs. Adams's problems by making and monitoring changes in her medications and instructing her on joint protection as she assumed new caregiving tasks. The team also helped her find a day center for Mr. Adams. The members of the team have fielded numerous calls from Mrs. Adams. As the events with her husband unfolded, Mrs. Adams had a serious flare-up of her arthritis. Team members enhanced their communication as they attempted to address Mrs. Adams's problems, fearing they would result in her incapacitation. The team added Mrs. Adams's name to the list of patients to discuss at their weekly care-planning meeting.

A large managed care organization had purchased the hospital that funded the clinic serving Mrs. Adams. The new administrator requested that the team physician attend a meeting to discuss the clinic operation. Subsequently, at the weekly care-planning meeting, the physician announced that the administrator was concerned about the clinic's financial status and that all of the clinics in the facility had to increase their efficiency. The administrator was particularly concerned with this clinic, because he decided it was using a team model that was resource-intensive and inherently inefficient. The administrator suggested that the team discontinue its weekly meeting to allow each team member to schedule four more patients for that day. The team members were stunned and were not sure how they would defend their team clinic operation.

As a response to the administrator's mandate, the clinic MSW and the NP wanted to meet with the administrator to defend the need for a team in the clinic. The team MD said that the managed care organization was measuring clinic productivity by the number of patient visits and that the clinic's productivity would be reflected in the team members' pay. He felt they should just accept the decision because they didn't have a chance of changing the philosophy of the new administration. Some of the team members were not sure if they wanted to continue working for the clinic and others decided to keep quiet for fear of losing their jobs.

The Westside Clinic in 2016

The administrators of the Westside Clinic have changed their thinking in relation to the team approach to care. The chief operating officer (COO) of the Westside Clinic was feeling pressure from the administrator of their admitting hospital because their rate of readmissions within 30 days was too high. The COO had applied for Medical Home certification.[2] The Patient-Centered Medical Home is a program sponsored by the National Committee for Quality Assurance and is focused on organizing primary care to emphasize care coordination and communication around the patient's needs and wants. The COO considered the medical home to be a way to improve care for patients with chronic and complex healthcare problems, and she was certain the team model would decrease hospital readmissions, increase clinic efficiency, and address the overuse of the emergency room. The COO established three primary care teams within the clinic. She had each team attend the TeamSTEPPS Program,[3] a one-day team development program offered by the Agency for Healthcare Quality.

A primary healthcare team—consisting of an RN case manager with a bachelor's degree (BSN), a family practitioner MD director, three NPs, two RNs with associate degrees, and two medical assistants (MA)—is operating at one of the three clinics. These providers comprise the core team within their clinic and have access by referral to a secondary team of providers including a social worker with a bachelor's degree (BSW), a psychologist (MS Psych), a physical therapist (LPT), an occupational therapist (OTR), a clinical pharmacist (PharmD), and a nutritionist with a bachelor's degree (RD). The secondary team is shared by the other two primary care clinics.

Although the medical director of the clinic requested a social worker as part of each core team, the COO refused, saying a social worker would be part of the secondary team and would be available to the core teams as needed. The COO also asked Human Resources to recruit a BSW rather than an MSW for the secondary team, because the BSW was less expensive, and she thought a BSW could do the job.

The primary team for the clinic holds daily "lightning" rounds to discuss the scheduled patients, focusing on patient problem lists and notes from referrals to secondary team members. One of the RNs has chronic back pain that affects her concentration during these meetings. She is reluctant to say anything because she is afraid of peer pressure from the other team members.

The secondary team members attend these "lightning" rounds when they don't have other duties that interfere with the meeting time. Sometimes team members send alternates from their respective departments. The core teams meet together every other week with an administrative officer to discuss the statistical tables that management analyzes from the data the team members enter into the electronic medical record (EMR) system. Sometimes these meetings consume time needed by providers to make follow-up phone calls to patients or delay staff referrals to other providers.

Management recently decreased time slots for patient visits to 20 minutes for intakes and 10 minutes for repeat visits. This angered some of the nursing staff, and, consequently, several RNs and an NP resigned, saying they could easily get jobs at the clinic down the street. The Westside Clinic responded by hiring two RNs who were recent graduates of the local technical college. The remaining NPs disapproved of the new hires because they did not have bachelor's degrees and they were unfamiliar with the EMR system.

Mr. and Mrs. Davis are typical patients seen in the medical home. Mr. Davis has Parkinson's disease with labile hypertension, decreasing mobility, and increasing memory loss. When he last picked up his prescriptions, the cost of his generic antihypertensive medicine was 500 percent more than it had been three months prior. Mr. Davis is not sure he wants to continue taking this medicine. Mr. Davis's primary physician recommended a new treatment, but Mr. Davis's insurer has refused to pay for it even after a letter of justification from the primary physician. The primary physician recommended that Mr. Davis challenge the decision of the insurance company, but Mr. and Mrs. Davis were too intimidated to appear before the panel of 12 reviewers.

Mrs. Davis has severe osteoarthritis in her spine and is worried she will need to quit her job as a hair stylist to care for her husband. She is not sure how she will be able to continue her health insurance, because the co-pays have increased in the past year and are beyond her ability to pay. She has started skipping appointments with her rheumatologist and goes to storefront clinics when she has a minor health problem. Mrs. Davis gets little joy from her life, and on her days off she prefers to stay in bed and ignore what she regards as her husband's too frequent pleas for help. Although she attended her husband's first clinic visit, she now calls special transport services for his clinic visits and lets him go by himself.

Similarities and Differences

In 2000, healthcare providers were often faced with defending their positions as they learned to cope with new systems of care and the pressure to increase efficiency and safety. In 2016, healthcare providers are more likely to go along with the administrative directives, leave their team, or leave the organization. Employees want to help people and do well when they feel supported by their organization.[4] However, a history of loosening corporate ties to employees that began in the 1980s has resulted in less employee loyalty to employers.[5] Turnover has become a major problem in larger cities where healthcare providers have greater choice of work environments.

Two seasoned nurses give their perspectives on the views of younger nurses in relation to authority and the team:

Kara: "I am a BSN and work on a hospital unit. If the team I worked on didn't function well and I had one or two patients where it didn't go well, I probably wouldn't stick around. I would get out. I did work at another hospital for two months, and I left because I didn't like the way they operated. I was used to how a smooth unit runs and that unit didn't, and it was reflected in patient care."

Tim: "I have been working for many years as the head nurse on a medical-surgical unit. Nurses in general are afraid of authority. You especially see it in the younger ones. And sometimes they don't speak up because they just don't care. Some people just want to do their job and go home."

Turnover wreaks havoc on developed healthcare teams unless they have systems in place to integrate new members into existing teams and are committed to the process.

On the surface, the way the Westside Clinic operated in 2000 and how it operated in 2016 didn't seem to be all that different. Both case examples present the interrelated clinical and social issues that continue to create complexity in health care. While many of the physical and emotional problems in patient care remain the same, the context of providing that care has changed. The themes that were building in 2000—e.g., increased efficiency, safety, cost effectiveness, and technology—have been magnified in 2016. With increasing corporatization, the way health care is delivered is in the hands of health system executives, healthcare administrators, insurers, informatics specialists, and pharmaceutical companies. Some of these entities have never cared for a patient in primary care, nor do they necessarily understand the capabilities of each health profession.

Corporate health care uses increasingly sophisticated methods to track data targeting quality of care, efficiencies, and system failures. This tracking is driven by the need to please shareholders and other major funding sources like Medicare and Medicaid. Rehospitalization within 30 days of discharge is one of the markers mandated by Medicare for certain cardiac and lung conditions. The fact that readmission is tied to reimbursement provides incentive for hospitals to change protocols with the hope of lowering their readmission rates. When news of one healthcare system's successful change in procedure is reported to reduce costs or readmission rates, other hospitals quickly follow. Unfortunately, in health care, unlike many businesses, each setting can be markedly dissimilar and adopting the same practices can produce unintended results.

One Size Does Not Fit All

The Cleveland Clinic is one hospital system that attempted to reduce readmissions by mandating a predischarge visit by a pharmacist to discuss medications. While this strategy decreased readmissions at the Cleveland Clinic, where most patients had health insurance and could afford their medications, it did not work at other Cleveland hospitals with more indigent populations, where they found their Medicare readmission fines increased after instituting this program.[6]

In another hospital system, Joye, a retired nurse, was being discharged from the hospital:

> **Joye:** "At 8 a.m. the day of discharge I told the charge nurse I wanted to be discharged early in the day so my husband could pick me up. The nurse said the pharmacist had to see me before I left. By 10 a.m. there was still no sign of the pharmacist. I called the nurse and she said the pharmacist would make rounds at 12:30. I said I was leaving. The pharmacist showed up five minutes later. But the thing was, I didn't need a pharmacist. None of my medicines had changed and I was well aware of how to take them."

These examples illustrate some of the problems with applying one solution to a wide variety of problems. Any of the hospitals mentioned could have patients with multiple acute and chronic health problems. Some patients might have mental health problems that interfere with their drug-taking behaviors. Some patients have caregivers who aren't able to care for them. Others might have problems paying for their medicines or transportation or mobility problems that interfered with obtaining their medicines; some might have early undiagnosed dementia, family members who were surreptitiously taking their opioid medicines, or, like Joye, not need a pharmacist consult.

The potential problems that relate to a patient taking medicine as prescribed are almost endless. Requiring a predischarge pharmacy visit for all patients might save some readmissions, but in the long run it is probably not the most cost-effective way to address the myriad of complex and often co-occurring problems that can occur. A comprehensive screening tool administered by a member of a well-developed and functioning IHT that includes a pharmacist, a nurse, and a social worker might be a more effective means of reducing readmissions. Using such a tool, any team member could decide which discipline, *if any*, should see a patient before discharge.

The same financial pressures that exist on the inpatient side of health care also exist in outpatient settings, and they affect the types of teams that are created. Administrators with either clinical or nonclinical backgrounds, who are removed from the ways healthcare providers, at different levels and from differing professions, are trained to think and to process information and to make important decisions in the way health care is delivered. Corporate pressures might dictate that a nurse with an associate's degree rather than a bachelor's degree, a behavioral health specialist with a social work practice certificate, or a social worker with a bachelor's degree rather than a master's degree will be assigned to a clinical setting.

Differing Levels of Understanding within the Professional Disciplines

Each professional discipline within health care has multiple certifications that represent different capacities for identifying problems, processing information, and making decisions. The meaning of these certifications is enhanced by the experiences clinicians have had in their professional fields. Managers and administrators who have not learned the meaning behind the certification levels of different disciplines or who have not been exposed to professionals' clinical problem solving might think a physician's assistant (PA) has the same training as an NP. They might not know the difference between an RN with an associate's degree, a BSN, or an MSN. They likely will not know the difference between a social worker with a practice certificate, a BSW or an MSW. They would also need to learn what different specialty certificates and licenses mean for each discipline.

The difference in the problem-solving abilities between different levels of providers is often underrated and misunderstood and is not normally taught in schools of management. Clinicians need to find ways to educate management about the capabilities within their respective disciplines. A useful team development exercise that includes healthcare professionals, managers, and administrators would be to ask each discipline to write and share activities that denote working to the top of their certification. They would additionally discuss activities that someone with a different type or level of expertise could accomplish more efficiently. It is particularly useful to openly discuss these issues in an early phase of team development.

Pressure to See More Patients

Economic pressures influence the number of patients a provider or team must see during a particular clinic and the amount of time in which each patient can be seen. This may mean increasing the number of patients seen while reducing patient contact time. While such decisions might not adversely affect some patients, others with complex needs will not receive the care they need in a timely manner, and, subsequently, they can become more burdensome on a healthcare system.

Mental health problems are pervasive, frequently invisible, and adversely affect our physical health. It takes exceptional expertise to recognize the difficulty of treating them and incorporating their treatment into current healthcare models that are biased toward physical symptom management. An interprofessional team approach to care is our best hope for accomplishing this feat in an era where the number of psychiatrists is declining. Administrators and funders need to be part of the discussion at every level to increase their understanding of how we can accomplish this union.

Healthcare system providers must understand that patients, their caregivers, and healthcare professionals with mental health problems have a unique way of slowing down the process of health care. Patients, family members, and/or providers can be hiding problems with alcohol abuse. Patients and family members and providers who are addicted to prescription or illegal drugs come in all sizes and occupations. Those who have been abused or who exhibit abusive behaviors, those with personality disorders or maladaptive behaviors consistent with personality disorders, and those with anxiety disorders all have different ways of presenting. Also, providers must have someone to turn to when they discover a member of their team is having or causing difficulty because of mental health problems. As providers are pressured to increase their patient loads and decrease the time they spend with patients, the more these mental health problems will be ignored and the more barriers they will create to the smooth delivery of health care.

Referrals to Other Providers

The art and skill of referring patients to other providers is taught as part of many residencies for healthcare professionals, particularly those in highly affiliated teaching and research institutions. However, healthcare practitioners who are new to their field might see referring patients to another provider as a reflection of their lack of knowledge. Or, perhaps they don't understand enough about what other providers do. Training that is intently focused on making us experts in our own profession can simultaneously cloud our perceptions of a problem and make us unaware of our single-minded deficits. Seasoned providers might view themselves as more skilled than they actually are.

A medical student who was preparing for a career in family practice was surprised when I told him that two of the most difficult things he would have to learn as a primary care physician were *whether* to refer a patient and *when* to refer a patient to another provider. He looked at me like I had just been diagnosed with a contagious disease. Some healthcare systems might discourage referrals to contain costs. Also some professionals might take a narcissistic pride in *doing it all* and not referring to other providers. A few years ago I was invited to address a workshop that included physicians and other healthcare professionals who were asked to function as a think tank for the newly passed U.S. Affordable Care Act. There were a number of prominent family physicians in the group. I repeated the message I had given to the medical student and added the following story.

> **John:** "I presented to my family physician with an ingrown toenail and asked for a referral to a podiatrist. My physician decided he could treat it by removing part of the toenail, saying it wasn't a problem as he could perform the debridement. After the procedure my toe was extremely sore and continued to bleed for weeks and I was unable to wear a shoe on that foot during one of the coldest winters on record. Six weeks later, as my toe was still sore and bleeding, I returned to my primary physician and he performed further debridement on the toe. When my toe still didn't heal I demanded to see a podiatrist."

After the workshop I shared a taxi to the airport with one of the primary care physician participants who elaborated on the difficult cases he had treated by himself. He said he prided himself in being able to meet each new challenge. It was clear he was chiding me for insinuating he could not handle any problem that came his way. I had no way to judge the quality of this physician's care and had not intended to insult his abilities. The fact that he participated in this brainstorming session for healthcare practice spoke to his qualifications. However, I wondered if the difficult procedures he was conquering at this later stage of his career were different from those he tackled at the beginning of his career.

Over time, all healthcare professionals continue to learn, increasing their skills, but at some point in their careers they sometimes perform activities and procedures that take them to the limit of their abilities. Their decisions could have multiple drivers, for example, a healthcare system that discourages referrals, a patient with limited insurance or endurance, ignorance of what other providers do, or perhaps the need for money to buy a new boat. At what point would the patient be better served by a provider making a referral or by conferring with a provider from another discipline? This is a difficult question that can best be answered after gaining an extensive knowledge of the skills and expertise of providers from other disciplines and specialties.

> **Katy:** "While skating I fell on my shoulder, heard a loud crack, and felt faint. Out of town at the time I bought a sling and stabilized my shoulder to avoid movement. Two days later and back at home, I scheduled an appointment with an NP in my primary care clinic. I told my story

emphasizing the loud crack I heard when I fell. After an X-Ray the NP diagnosed me with a bruised bursa saying I did not need to use the sling. I told the NP I thought there was something more wrong than a bruised bursa. The NP made a referral to physical therapy.

A week later the PT evaluated my shoulder and after two treatments said she did not think I had a bruised bursa, and was concerned because I was not responding to treatment. I felt something was very wrong and asked the PT if I should see an orthopedic surgeon. She said the surgeon would not order an MRI till the swelling was down so she didn't see the point. She continued treatments for three more weeks while saying I was losing function. I again requested to see an orthopedic surgeon. The PT said she needed to refer back to the NP, but would word her note so the NP would order an MRI and likely make a referral.

Results of the MRI showed a shredded labrum and, on exam, the surgeon also diagnosed a fractured humerus saying I should have been placed in a sling, and not sent to PT."

In her initial contact with the NP, it was apparent Katy knew something was terribly wrong, but she was unable to verbalize her concerns in language the NP readily accepted. Perhaps the NP had been previously chastised for inappropriate referrals by the orthopedic surgeon. It is unknown why Katy's concerns were initially ignored.

The stories of John and Katy are examples of the thousands of everyday problems confronting those who work in health care. The knowledge a practitioner must have to make the multiple decisions on whether or how to treat and/or to make timely consultations and appropriate referrals is enormous and highly underestimated. Unless providers have established relationships and appropriate referral patterns with providers from other disciplines, patients might not receive timely care. It takes time and opportunities provided by healthcare administrators for providers to learn the extent of their own knowledge and limitations relative to other professionals in their system and beyond.

Amanda: "I was marching in a parade and tripped over a spectator's extended leg. I was taken to the emergency department (ED) with facial lacerations and a very painful knee. The ED surgeon said I had fractured my left kneecap in six places and thought I should have reconstructive surgery. He said the surgery was very complex and he felt there were only four surgeons in the state who were capable of saving my knee. All of them were outside the jurisdiction of my network healthcare provider. The ED surgeon submitted a request and justification to my network insurance provider. He also intervened when the request was initially denied. Someone from my network provider finally approved one of the four surgeons suggested by the ED surgeon. Two weeks later I had successful surgery. I was so grateful that the ED surgeon went above and beyond to do this for me. I also appreciated that the ED staff kept me informed along the way."

The successful outcome of Amanda's case required knowledge of the skills of individual physicians from different specialties and subspecialties. If the ED surgeon had little knowledge of the skills of the surgeons in his region, the outcome would likely have been less satisfactory for Amanda.

Difficulties Inherent in Requesting Help

Providers, support staff, and patients encounter situations daily in which they try to solve a complex problem with only part of the knowledge necessary to do so. After multiple attempts at addressing a problem with limited success, a clinician might realize that the solution requires knowledge that she does not have and does not have time to acquire. Patients and administrators are a large and often ignored part of the complex care equation. When a patient feels she is not being helped, she might seek out another provider or simply give up trying to address her problem. An administrator with inadequate knowledge of the capacities of each healthcare profession cannot make sound decisions about allocation of resources.

In clinical healthcare settings uncertainty is common and consults are often in the best interests of the patient. For practitioners, the search for additional knowledge might be from another colleague from the same profession. Or a professional might seek the help of a provider from another profession, an administrator, or a member of the support staff, especially if the provider has established a relationship with that person. If a provider does not know or have a relationship with the provider they are consulting, the result might not be as expected.

Most providers have stories about asking a physician for help and being rebuked or rebuffed. Physicians also have stories of consulting with another physician they don't personally know and being chastised.

Ned: "As an ED physician I needed to consult another physician to obtain permission for an MRI study on a patient. The hospital made that requirement to assure the ED docs were using MRIs appropriately. A new surgeon was on call, and so I called him and welcomed him to the community and introduced myself as the medical director of the ED. I said I appreciated having a neurosurgeon in town, and proceeded to tell him about the

> patient and when I finished he said, 'Just because you have a surgeon on call doesn't mean you call me for every little thing that happens in the ED.' I said, I have never spoken to you before, and this is how you talk to me. He then proceeded to talk about the patient but nothing he said was helpful to me. I got off the phone and vented saying he needed charm school. I then called another surgeon. The real tragedy was the unfriendly surgeon only lasted a month and a half in our system. It is very costly to hire someone who doesn't work out. Also, if a surgeon doesn't work out, chances are he isn't doing a lot of surgery and that is also costly."

Poor responses from someone we count on to provide more information can affect a provider's willingness to reach out and collaborate when joint problem solving is a necessity. Establishing effective relationships takes time and can be difficult in a system where progress is measured in numbers of procedures performed.

Sometimes an informal collaboration with another provider is the most efficient way to solve a problem, but without a functioning team it can be a problem to contact another colleague and get a quick response to a question. There is often a lag time or the consult report does not appear in the chart in a location where it is readily available to the referring provider. If we try to informally collaborate, the system might not support that collaboration. When similar and/or complex problems arise frequently, those we ask for help might become irritated or resentful that we are asking so much of their time when they have their own jobs to do. Thus, the consultation process may be inefficient for certain problems that require a more formal team effort with established expectations, goals, procedures, and responsibilities.

Motivation among team members to practice teamwork plays a large role in whether or not a team works. Some healthcare providers begin working on teams, because they realize that they cannot provide care alone for some patients and see it as a better way to practice. Other providers might be forced by their supervisor to join a team. Unless the team they join functions well and has processes in place to bring new team members along or to examine team issues, the health professional who is forced into a team setting will likely be dissatisfied and have even less of a reason to engage. Healthcare professionals will prefer to perform their work the way they were trained and, without comprehensive training in teamwork, will likely place little value on it.

Until recently, most clinicians' training has been insular within their respective professional school. While students, they might have attended a few lectures or even engaged in a few clinical rotations with students from other professions, but the curriculum from one profession was generally not integrated with that of other professional schools. Professional students were not commonly taught a foundation for either building or working on sustained well-functioning interprofessional healthcare teams. As those professionals continue in the workforce they will need to be exposed to role models and continuing education to change their behaviors. Even now, the interprofessional training of students of the health professions is not fully integrated on most campuses. It will take many years for the completion of this ideal.

Attempts have been made to teach interprofessional concepts to students. However, engaging in interprofessional didactic and group experiences are not the same as functioning on an interprofessional team. In our experience, if health profession trainees don't experience interprofessional team concepts in actual practice on well-functioning healthcare teams, their use of team knowledge rapidly diminishes. The health professions' students must also participate in interprofessional teamwork during a significant part of their education. Students should be exposed to IHTs early in their training with the level of exposure increasing as students approach their clinical practice. Exposure to administrative staff as team members needs to be part of the student experience. Students readily recognize incongruities. If students perceive a lack of value or little appreciation for IHTs or see that their role models do not practice interprofessional teamwork, it is reasonable to expect that students will neither value IHTs nor choose to practice in them.

In an effort to contain costs, administrators might turn to lesser-trained providers to accomplish many healthcare tasks. Providing interprofessional educational and training experiences for healthcare providers such as nursing assistants, licensed practical nurses (LPNs), RNs with associate degrees, and social workers with certificates who do not earn at least a bachelor's degree in their professional field is an extremely difficult problem for administrators. There is very little, if any, time in their training programs for interprofessional education. This leaves a large gap in IHT formation that administrators will need to fill. Administrators need to work with educators in finding ways to train these individuals so they feel enabled as partners in teamwork. Programs like TeamSTEPPS can help in this regard. However, these individuals need time to participate in such programs and to practice what they learn.

Once healthcare professionals are in practice settings, they will perform according to what they have learned in their training and adapt that knowledge to conform to conditions in their work environment. Even healthcare professionals with solid backgrounds in how IHTs function will lose their skills if the organizational culture and administrative staff neither value interprofessional teamwork nor provide resources for team development and maintenance.

Summary

The corporatization of health care has precipitated a movement toward efficiency, accuracy, and safety. However, the data and methodologies used to propel those goals may be insufficient to achieve them, especially in the primary care of patients with complex problems requiring an interprofessional teamwork approach. If health care is to achieve efficiencies, it cannot ignore the complexities of addressing both physical and mental health problems in patients, caregivers, and even in practitioners. If insurers and healthcare administrators do not understand the complexities inherent in interprofessional teamwork, teams will not thrive; or if they thrive they will not be able to achieve efficiency and effectiveness. If the business of health care does not take a comprehensive long-term view in its evaluation process, it will not realize that developing IHTs takes time, but can ultimately save money in turnover costs, decreases in repeat hospital admissions, and more accurate care. Without these realizations, IHTs will not be valued and will not survive. Administrators, educators, and healthcare professionals must work together in a mutual teaching and learning environment with the goal of sharing their expertise in solving the complexities of health care in a business-driven environment.

Questions for Discussion

1. What activities denote working to the top of your certification?
2. How can administrators and managers be most helpful to the team process?
3. What are some situations that occurred during your healthcare career in which asking for help from other disciplines might have produced a better outcome?
4. In what ways can administrators, educators, and practitioners work together to establish a common understanding of IHTs?

3

Healthcare Teams and Business Teams: A Mix of Assumptions and Values

Healthcare professions attract some of the best and brightest students. As a group, healthcare professionals are caring people who value giving good patient care. Their goal is to provide patients the help they need no matter the obstacles. During the past three decades, business professionals have become an integral part of the healthcare model and healthcare teams. Healthcare professionals have generally accepted the mandates that corporatization has brought, not only because openly complaining is not part of their DNA, but also because they love what they do and generally just want to perform their jobs.

However, the business model emanates from traditional economic theory and, unlike the ideal standard value model of healthcare professionals, the business model is based on "an abstract caricature of self-interest."[1] Since the middle of the 20th century, a goal of business has been to broaden this value system to include social and community responsibility.[2] However, economics remains a large part of the business ideal, and, depending on the ebb and flow of monetary resources, it exerts pressure on healthcare professionals to increase their efficiency. The incorporation of the business model into health care directly affects how healthcare professionals perceive their practice and their roles on IHTs.

There is no denying that inserting business professionals into health care has brought efficiencies to practice. However, if healthcare administrators and funders do not have a thorough understanding of how healthcare professionals are trained and how they think differently from those who are trained in business, the added value of the business model may eventually be detrimental to the patient. The richness of business philosophies must be coupled with the richness and ethical mandates of the varied schools of healthcare practice in a way that enhances care for the patient. This can only be accomplished through high-level interprofessional dialogue that integrates the difficult issues of very complex patients.

Integrating solutions for the difficult and interacting problems of patients is the strength of IHTs that are not just assemblages of individuals from different professions. IHTs are complex and often paradoxical entities that sometimes seem to defy understanding. Team situations that appear easy and straightforward are not. Individuals who preach teamwork are not always willing to support it. Teams that seem to be developed and well-functioning may be full of camouflaged chaos. And, teams that seem chaotic and dysfunctional may actually be creating unique solutions to vexing problems.

As clinicians begin to interact more closely with other care providers, they realize that providers from different disciplines have philosophies that differ from theirs. Team members find it difficult to address the professional values, language differences, inevitable conflict issues, different problem-solving styles, and systems issues that teamwork brings. Without a context for decision making, it is difficult for healthcare providers who are from diverse fields with uniquely focused goals and different problem-solving methodologies to dialogue effectively for the benefit of the patient. This is why complex healthcare situations require formal structures and processes that efficiently and effectively use the talents of professionals from different disciplines.

We believe that you can effectively use only what you truly understand. It follows that if healthcare and business professionals do not fully understand IHTs, they will be able to neither create efficient teams nor defend them to administrators and funding sources. Team members who are hired to work on an IHT often contribute to future decisions on hiring additional team members. If those hired have not had sufficient training in interprofessional teamwork, a cycle of incompetence can be created that may be devastating for a team. Hiring either healthcare or business professionals with little to no training in interprofessional teamwork can signal to administrators that IHTs are inefficient or not necessary for a particular clinic.

In this chapter we will begin to explore a common understanding of IHTs by reviewing some definitions of teams. We will also review some of the different attributes of IHTs in a variety of settings. Additionally, we will address some of the differences and similarities that exist between philosophies of IHTs and business teams such as self-directed work teams (SDWTs) or project teams.

Definitions of Teams and Groups: A Muddle of Terminology

"Let's get a team to work on this!" "Let's call ourselves a team!" "We make the best team!" "The power of teamwork!" Since working together is a part of the human experience, the simple word *team* has become a catchword for a group of people who are designated as working together in some capacity (e.g., teaching team, business team, healthcare team, sports team, project team, self-directed team). The word *team* is commonly applied to many different types of teams and methods of working with others.

In speaking of teams, we might not appreciate that within health care, different types of teams have unique cultural attributes. Over time, primary care teams, surgical teams, home care teams, rehabilitation teams, geriatrics teams, and mental health teams have developed similar but separate cultures to meet specific needs of their patients. Even IHTs in similar settings are not necessarily alike. When healthcare providers receive their training in one team setting and end up working in another, they may be surprised to find that there are major team differences between the two settings. IHTs also take on unique characteristics, and these characteristics change over time as an IHT either develops or regresses in its growth pattern.

The term *team* is used almost universally to describe groups of people who work together in some capacity. When an entity is too complex to understand, simplifying its use affords people a way to cope with it. One of the drawbacks to simplifying the expression *team* is assuming understanding when the concerned parties are discussing different entities. These assumptions are common between healthcare providers and are becoming more common between providers and administrators.

It is equally widespread for physicians to equate the term *healthcare team* with a group of MDs from the same or different specialties. Health professionals who work in the same unit but have very little contact with each other may refer to themselves as a team or be referred to as a team. Administrators tend to think in terms of project teams and short-term task teams. Patients may or may not have their own concept of team. Additionally, the cultures inherent in business models introduce a different set of values from those of healthcare models. For example, the culture in an information technology department might be much more informal than that in a finance department.

Healthcare Team Attributes

Healthcare teams could have an almost infinite number of variables. A team might have 2 members or 20; be temporary or permanent; provide ongoing care or merely perform assessments; be recently assembled, long term, or a mix of the two; contain all experts or all generalists; have all members of the same discipline or of many disciplines; or have members who are solely assigned to one team or to multiple teams. Within this broad context there is an array of potential meanings that render the term *team* unusable if it is not accompanied by a specific definition.

Healthcare teams have been described as multidisciplinary, interdisciplinary, interprofessional, cross disciplinary, polydisciplinary, pandisciplinary, transdisciplinary, interactive, and virtual. Unfortunately, these terms are often used interchangeably to refer to team. Perhaps it is because the word *team* encompasses so many variables that it is often reduced to the least common denominator.

In an effort to determine the extent of the problem of misusing the term *healthcare team* in the field of geriatrics, Drinka and Ray[3] conducted a cross-sectional review of the geriatrics literature for any articles that related to healthcare teams. The review covered the years 1982, 1986, and 1990. This review revealed that although most articles were descriptive, with the intent of teaching general geriatrics, the teams were not well described. Physician-directed patient outcome studies of acute care consult teams appeared to be increasing without adequate descriptors of the independent variable, which was the team.

Consult teams may have been the least likely type of team to benefit elderly patients, and yet, in the early 1990s, these acute care teams (without description) represented the majority being studied in the geriatrics literature. These articles were in journals directed to MDs, the discipline with the most influence in healthcare systems. After reviewing the more recent literature focused on healthcare teams, it is clear the term *interprofessional* has been widely accepted to describe teams with providers from multiple disciplines. However, this has not solved the problems with misuse of terms; neglecting to specify the attributes of the team under study; or using team descriptors interchangeably. A notable exception to this is a book chapter by Steffen and colleagues.[4]

Overgeneralization of the team concept might also cause team members to assume if you merely assemble a group of nice people, team building will not be necessary. It can also lead administrators to believe that one or two days of team building will be sufficient to develop functional inter-professional teams. Healthcare professionals support those generalizations when they assert that they are busy with the important work of caring for people and do not have additional time for team building and team maintenance, which they view as less important than delivering health care. Healthcare systems contribute further to these overgeneralizations because funding for healthcare services is generally based on number of patients seen or on procedures completed. If administrators and professionals do not see immediate results from team maintenance activities, they do little to promote them.

Professionals who work well with one or two other professionals may behave very differently in a group. Identifying a group of people and calling them a team does not mean that they function well or at all as a team. Providing several days of team training to professionals does not ensure they will continue to function as a team. Healthcare and business professionals can also behave very differently in a short-term team than they do in a long-term team. And, since most health professionals have been trained to function autonomously, some might have difficulty in any collaborative team environment.

It is easy to imagine a virtual team that communicates primarily by telephone, e-mail, texting, and/or satellite hookups. It might be more difficult to imagine a well-functioning IHT that has first agreed on processes and structures for communication, developed a pattern of leadership and trust, and established methods for evaluation. Maintaining this groundwork for a well-functioning and effective IHT takes time and collective effort. That is the "stuff" of teams that is rarely spoken of and is often left to chance. When team maintenance is left to chance, teams usually get into trouble. When teams experience trouble, they either obtain help, limp along until they dissolve, or become so inefficient that the organization eventually "reorganizes" and puts them out of their misery.

Members of IHTs and business teams frequently harbor images of the teams (past and present) on which they have served. Negative and positive experiences are remembered at both conscious and subconscious levels and undoubtedly affect how members engage or don't engage with new teammates. For example, imagine an MD who had worked well with a bachelor's-prepared RN (BSN) who had specialty training in diabetes care on a previous team wanting to hire an RN for another team. The team member from management was getting pressure to cut costs and, being unaware of the difference in training, decided to hire an RN who had just graduated with an associate degree in nursing. The MD might be surprised by the discrepancy in the knowledge between the two RNs and blame the new RN for a deficiency of knowledge.

Images of teams are also a reflection of interpersonal experiences—past and present. These interpersonal experiences with family, friends, and acquaintances lay the groundwork for the way team members view themselves in relation to a team and how quickly they assimilate into the team. If a professional always assumed a leadership role with her siblings, she might naturally assume a leadership role on a team. If a professional has a history of introversion or of making decisions alone, it might take that person longer to develop trust in the team.

A Definition of Interprofessional Healthcare Team

Since the function and structure of an IHT can have an impact on the type of care that is delivered, studies involving healthcare teams should contain adequate descriptors of the team variable. This is important because different types of teams have different costs and benefits and produce different outcomes. Another reason why it is important to use the terminology of teams correctly—or at least to define the terminology that is being used—is because a common understanding helps people communicate more efficiently with greater accuracy. In a field that has been so misunderstood, use of commonly understood terminology is critical to gaining credibility.

For the purposes of this book an IHT is defined as follows:

> An IHT integrates a group of individuals with diverse training and backgrounds who work together as an identified unit or system. Team members consistently collaborate to solve patient problems that are too complex to be solved by one discipline or many disciplines in sequence. In order to provide care as efficiently as possible, an IHT creates formal and informal structures that encourage collaborative problem solving. Team members determine the team's mission and common goals, work interdependently to define and treat patient problems, and learn to accept and capitalize on disciplinary differences, differential power, and overlapping roles. To accomplish these they share leadership that is appropriate to the presenting problem and promote the use of differences for confrontation and collaboration. They also use collected data and team member observations to evaluate the team's work and its development.

The concept of a functional unit is particularly important because it allows for a continuously evolving core operation for evaluation, feedback, and improvement.

At the most basic level, teamwork relies on the ability of team members to communicate with one another. If practitioners are not sure who is on the team and they are a member of the team, it is difficult to know what, how, when, or with whom to communicate. Also, if the team has not agreed on what needs to be communicated, there will be disparate views about what information to pass on to other members—which members and in what format. The more that IHTs leave cross discipline communication to chance or restrict it to formal occasions, the more likely it is that communication will not happen when the complexity and seriousness of a situation call for it.

Differing Cultures of Interprofessional Healthcare Teams

Discussing cultures of any kind can be dangerous as one may be accused of stereotyping. However, in our experience there appear to be differences in the way various types of IHTs develop and in the values that they hold about how to behave. Just as populations in different parts of a city or areas of a country develop unique ways of behaving, in health care different cultures emerge in various subspecialty departments. Also, IHTs in a variety of healthcare settings may attract certain personality types and people who share unique goals and values for delivering care.

Primary Care Teams

Primary care IHTs tend to attract individuals who specialize in variety and who like following patients on a long-term basis. Primary care teams tend to have fewer core disciplines, usually physicians, nurse practitioners, physician assistants (MDs/NPs/PAs), RNs or licensed practical nurses (LPNs), and medical or nursing assistants (MAs). Some primary care teams also include a mental health worker like a social worker or clinical psychologist. Having a greater variety of disciplines as part of a core team enables the primary care team to increase the accuracy of decisions. However, including more disciplines on the team may not be economically feasible. In these situations, it is critical for members of the primary care team to learn the skills and levels of training of other disciplines. This enables the team to make accurate and timely referrals, bringing other disciplines into their team as consultants or temporary members. Key skills for primary care providers include knowing what to treat, how much to treat, and when to refer.

It is also vital for primary care teams to learn skills in interteam communication. In some primary care settings, there is a trend toward hiring less skilled workers (e.g., MAs or LPNs) to perform more of the work that gets reimbursed, like reviewing medications, blood pressure, and weight monitoring. However, if the team does not establish procedures and training for communication between different levels of providers, members may have difficulty knowing their limits and when and how to use the skills of the other team members. In this case, the team may be unable to reap the real economic benefits of having multiple levels of providers. For example, if an MA's job is to review the patient's medications but he or she cannot pronounce the names of medications correctly, the patient might be unlikely to respond when the MA asks for the patient's primary concerns.

Geriatrics Teams

IHTs in geriatric settings have the same long-term focus as primary care teams but might assume a slower pace because of the nature of their patients. The primary focus of IHTs in geriatrics is evaluating and treating older frail patients with complex and interacting physical and psychosocial problems. They concentrate on helping the patient achieve and sustain quality of life and focus less on curing all the patient's problems. Because of the complexity of their patients, geriatric teams usually have a greater mix of highly trained team members from different professional disciplines, for example, social workers with master's degrees (MSWs) instead of bachelor's degrees (BSWs). Healthcare providers who receive team training in geriatrics do not assume that the MD/NP/PA must be "the leader" of the team. They learn to develop many leaders with different leadership skills and to promote different types of leadership where and when it is needed.

Unfortunately, retaining a highly developed IHT has not always been the case for geriatrics teams because administrators sometimes assigned professionals who were problem employees in other departments to the most chronic care teams where administrators thought they could do the least harm. This practice is changing as administrators realize the value in using a well-trained IHT to keep frail and chronically ill patients from repeat hospitalizations.

In long-term care settings for geriatric patients, team members may be unskilled workers or lesser-skilled professionals. This presents a problem for teamwork, because in a setting where team members other than the MD should take over leadership roles, team members may not have the skills to do so, and either weak or autocratic leadership may emerge. Geriatrics IHTs, like primary care teams, do not necessarily take the time to work on team process issues. However, when skilled professionals are assigned to work in geriatric IHTs, they have the capacity to create teams of greatness.

Rehabilitation Teams

Rehabilitation teams focus on intense treatment and rapid turnover. IHTs in rehabilitation departments usually have MDs, physical therapists (PTs), PT assistants, occupational therapists (OTs), and OT assistants. Depending on the setting, they might also have MDs who specialize in rehabilitation medicine, RNs with various levels of training, and speech pathologists. Leadership of the teams can range from MDs in more acute care settings to physical therapy assistants in chronic care rehabilitation settings. Decisions on formal leadership are increasingly made by management and based on cost and availability of a particular professional discipline.

Although rehabilitation teams may have multiple levels of providers, team members are usually well trained in their discipline-specific tasks and are used to working autonomously. In acute and subacute settings, the MD is commonly the clinical leader of the team. In rehabilitation clinic settings, practitioners from different levels of one discipline perform tasks that are defined by a team member from a higher level of that discipline, such as a PT directing a PT assistant or an OT directing an OT assistant. Each team member performs tasks that are limited by their professional training, although team members may informally share some tasks. Team members report their findings to the team and the MD or other leader makes final decisions on difficult questions of treatment.

Surgical Teams

IHTs in surgical settings are fast-paced, highly integrated units with patient safety as their number one priority. Surgical teams include surgeons, nurse or physician anesthetists, NPs/PAs, RNs of varying training, MAs/LPNs, and PTs or other therapists related to the specialty procedures. In the past 16 years, surgical IHTs have worked hard to increase their team safety procedures. Surgical IHTs usually focus on a specific patient problem and view their relationship with the patient as short term.

Surgeons rely on well-trained professional team members like NPs/PAs or PTs to perform pre- and postscreenings on patients during clinic visits. They also rely on MAs/LPNs to perform some tasks, such as suture removal and medication reviews. Other team members who assist in surgery may be more closely attached to a surgery center and will likely work with multiple surgeons. Because of the rapid turnover from inpatient or surgery center patient to outpatient status, surgical teams need good communication with team members in the surgical clinics. Accurate communications between team members from surgery clinics and team members from surgery centers can be difficult to establish and sustain.

Specialty Teams

Specialty IHTs are formed to address chronic, complex, and high-cost problems, like hypertension, medication management, pain, stroke, chronic obstructive pulmonary disease, or diabetes. Specialty IHTs include professionals with special knowledge of the problem being addressed, such as an MD, NP, or PA; RN specialists who often have master's degrees; pharmacist; and dietitian for a diabetes clinic; or MD/NP/PA, MSW, RN, OT, and speech therapist for a stroke clinic. Other disciplines may be included in these teams depending on the problem or focus. Team members usually work closely together in an interactive manner, with the primary focus of controlling the main problem and keeping the patient as independent as possible. Specialty IHTs have varying leadership but are often formally led by an RN, NP, or PA.

Surgical and other specialty teams may have benefited the most from the quality improvement (QI) movement because they are more narrowly focused than other settings like primary care and geriatrics, making it easier to establish and measure definable goals.

Mental Health Teams

IHTs in mental health settings are comprised of psychiatrists, psychologists, MSWs, RNs with mental health specialties, and other counselors. They focus on the emotional aspects of patients, relying on consults from MDs/NPs/PAs and allied health professionals if problems arise that are not of a mental health nature. Of all team types, mental health team members are the best trained to address the process issues of teams. This is both an asset and a liability. They have the capacity to ensure that the team achieves a high level of functioning. However, because they are so skilled at understanding psychological interactions, they are also skilled at using them to avoid conflict situations that could propel the team to greater heights of function.

IHTs that specialize in mental health problems value decision making by consensus and will take time to ensure that every member is heard. In making sure that everyone on the team has an equal say, they may get bogged down in values and ethical dilemmas, extending the time for resolving clinical issues. Because of their slower and more studied pace and the fact that team members are trained to look for emotional causes to problems, IHTs in mental health settings sometimes have difficulty communicating with other types of medically focused healthcare teams. This can compromise the ability of mental health providers to recognize medical problems at an early stage. Additionally, IHTs focusing on mental health need to work on increasing their efficiency in decision making without compromising their ability to confront team conflict.

Home Care and Chronic Care Treatment Teams

Home care and chronic care IHTs might differ according to mission, and new team models are continually emerging. Generally, home care teams are comprised of several levels of nursing staff (e.g., NPs, RNs at various levels, LPNs, and MAs). Home care teams also may have PTs, OTs, BSWs/MSWs, speech pathologists, chore workers, and personal care workers. An MD usually functions in a consultant role as medical director and likely attends some administrative team meetings. Because the team's work is physically diffused in the community, the professionals on this type of team are frequently self-directed thinkers who spend much of their time making autonomous decisions. While this trait is helpful in many situations these team members encounter, it can be an impediment when they are working with very complex patient conditions. Team members are used to communicating via phone and computer and in crisis situations rapid communication is essential.

IHTs in home care settings have a critical need to develop systems for describing problems in an integrative manner and for rapid communication on complex and unstable patients. And although these teams can benefit from the technology of computers and cell phones, they are teams that need to be highly developed and whose members need to be trained in the process skills of communication. When there are conflicts between members on home care teams, it is all too easy to ignore them until they become problems that can devastate a team. An additional problem in home care teams is the need to develop trust between different levels of providers with whom members may have little in-person contact.

Despite the varied cultures that exist in IHTs from different settings, all IHTs have some things in common, that is, a strong desire to help patients and a need for interprofessional team development and maintenance activities. It is critical for all IHTs to focus on their strengths and to address their weaknesses on an ongoing basis. The organization must allow them time for periodic review of their team process and functions. An organization's managers must also help ensure that teams are evaluating their function in line with the team and the organization's goals for care.

Differences and Similarities between Interprofessional Health Care Teams and Self-Directed Work Teams in Business

It is important to look at self-managed or self-directed work teams (SDWTs) in business settings because they have a history that is comparable to IHTs. Also, most of the administrators of healthcare organizations have been trained in a business culture and have brought that culture into health care. Successful SDWTs have interdependent members, a shared goal/mission, a climate of trust, open/honest communication, a sense of belonging, consensus decision making, and participative leadership. Diversity is valued as an asset, and creativity and risk taking are encouraged. A SDWT develops the ability to self-correct by examining its processes and practices.[5]

Differences

IHTs differ from SDWTs in business by virtue of their members, definition of consumer, and nature of their "product." Many of the theories developed for work teams in non–healthcare settings present problems when applied to IHTs (e.g., the primary focus of business teams on efficiency and ultimately the bottom line; the presence of physicians on IHTs; the patient's relationship to the healthcare team; and the uncertain nature of physical and mental health, which makes the end product in health care difficult to measure).

Primary Focus on Cost and the Bottom Line

Healthcare professionals are trained to put the patient's welfare first. This is in stark contrast to the primary focus of business teams on emphasizing efficiency, decreasing costs, and creating returns for investors. This is one of the greatest differences between the culture of healthcare and business professionals. The issue of cost of care and a patient's ability to pay for health care can present monumental ethical dilemmas that healthcare providers have been ill prepared to address. And yet, health care has increasingly become a cost-conscious business. Healthcare providers have been drawn into that business largely through the quality improvement and lean manufacturing movements that were adopted by business to improve efficiencies in manufacturing.

The Institute for Healthcare Improvement (IHI) adopted the principles of quality improvement and applied them to health care. The five focus areas of IHI include using improvement science to drive work, empowering the patient and family to be true partners in their care, ensuring patient safety, driving affordable health care through quality improvement, and improving population health while reducing cost per capita. On the IHI website (IHI.org), they endorse TeamSTEPPS, a program created by the Department of Health and Human Services Agency for Healthcare Research and Quality (AHRQ) and the Department of Defense's military health system. The program consists of a tool kit for evidence-based team training and implementation, focusing on teamwork skills like communication.[6] It is intended to optimize interprofessional team performance and outcomes. The impetus for TeamSTEPPS was the Institute of Medicine's call for "interdisciplinary team training programs that incorporate proven methods for team management to prevent medical errors."

Of the five focus areas of IHI, the ones that appear to have influenced development of TeamSTEPPS and IHT development have been "driving affordable health care" and "patient safety." The program is heavily influenced by sports metaphors and business terminology. The integration of the business model into healthcare team curriculum appears to be very strong. The TeamSTEPPs curriculum is now being taught in schools of nursing. How much this has narrowed the inherent dissimilarities between economically driven business models and the patient-focused care models imbued in the training programs for professional healthcare providers is unknown.

Presence of Physicians and Other Autonomous Disciplines

IHTs are unique among work teams because health care requires involvement by MDs. In the United States, by tradition, MDs have the highest level of training and the most ascribed power, and, in the medical literature, they have been referred to as the formal team leaders.[7] Although physicians are learning more about distributive leadership in their training, members of less developed IHTs might still defer to them as the leader of the team. In many areas of health care, NPs/PAs have become independent practitioners relatively free from physician influence. In the past 16 years, it has become commonplace for PTs and pharmacists to hold doctorates. These highly trained providers are also positioning themselves as formal team leaders. Alternatively, they often choose to practice autonomously.

The relative high status of MDs and other highly trained healthcare providers, coupled with the learned expectations of other health professionals, establishes a double bind for IHTs. A continued expectation of MD leadership plays out in several ways. Despite the fact that some MDs and other highly trained healthcare providers may attempt to incorporate certain expectations of leadership into the team process, they often have limited time and heavy commitments that prevent them from effectively executing their presumed leadership roles. The team's members may also expect that an MD or other highly trained team member will assume a formal leadership role when that individual has no intention of doing so.

Patients often complicate this game of chance, with expectations that their MD/NP/PA makes their healthcare decisions. However, the nature of a patient's problems might require team members who are not primary providers to assume leadership roles. IHTs and SDWTs have members from autonomous disciplines with specialized education and unique languages. Separatist attitudes that exist among professionals from different disciplines, especially in times of stress, may promote rejection of leaders from other disciplines and impede openness, innovation, and constructive confrontation in addressing complex problems. Patients with complex problems get caught between these highly trained disciplines when healthcare professionals are not working within an IHT. If a highly trained nonphysician provider makes a mistake, the patient will likely cut off contact and seek out a physician.

Patient's Relationship to the IHT

Although patients are not necessarily part of an ongoing team, they are central to the team's role and, unlike customers in a business model, often have to be invited to participate in their care decisions. Patients increasingly want to play a role in decisions that relate to their health. However, patients' desires for involvement in their IHT are as complex as their health care. Like team members who simplify team concepts, patients might try to oversimplify their health care so they can better understand it.

Many healthcare systems allow patients to ask questions of health providers through their Internet portals. However, it can become burdensome for providers to field questions that might be inappropriate for electronic communication or take time to answer when the provider is not reimbursed for the time. Many healthcare systems also limit access by patients to a specific number of inquiries. Also, despite this additional mechanism for access, patients are generally uncertain how to be involved as a member of their IHT. It is important for IHTs to provide guidelines for patient involvement in their team care. Members of an IHT might also have to teach patients how to most effectively interact with providers. This process involves a willingness to teach and learn by team members and assurances of understanding from the patient.

Understanding the sometime conflicting interplay of patient emotion and intellect is at the heart of the IHT's work. However, patients may not want to listen to the complex interactions that are potentiated by life and death therapies that may be required for their care. The most critical and difficult interactions often come at a time when a patient is least likely to understand and is the most vulnerable to being misunderstood by the team.

Uncertain Nature of Physical and Mental Health

Patient's bodies are not mechanized, and, unlike most businesses, choosing a healthcare procedure is not a sum-certain game. Patients are not customers in a business sense, and this presents ethical issues for the IHT. A patient might be well-informed and know what he wants. However, given the variables in the human body, that patient might not end up with what he wants. Another patient might be very well-informed and not have the emotional stability to make a reasonable decision. Other patients might be ill-informed and not understand their conditions or how their conditions relate to other maladies they might have. Sometimes patients are presented with an array of unpalatable options. They cannot decide what they want or what might be best for them. Also, illness can block even an assertive and well-informed person's ability to obtain or absorb the information necessary to make good healthcare decisions.

The uncertainty inherent in the outcomes of health care adds weight to the ethical dilemmas that face the IHT. In general, health is an extremely complex entity. Physical symptoms are mediated by psychological states and vice versa. Many conditions are interacting and have no easy cures. In addition, what one person sees as a cure might not be seen as a cure by another.

The following cases highlight some disparate views about surgical outcomes.

> **Mary:** "I had surgery on my eyes to correct my vision. For one week my vision greatly improved so I could see 20/20 out of each eye. The surgeon declared my case to be a success. However, within 6 weeks my vision deteriorated so I had difficulty seeing well out of either eye. I kept making appointments with the surgeon who would check my eyes. However he never acknowledged the surgery was a failure and did not provide me with any alternatives."

> **Ken:** "I had laparoscopic surgery on my back and was featured in a television piece about a successful new method of surgery. Within a month my leg pain and numbness had returned. Although the hospital marketing department considered the surgery a success, in my mind it turned out not to be."

Advances in healthcare remedies and technology seem to come almost daily. And, for every change, there is a potential interaction with an existing remedy or technology. There are few places in business where daily decisions in an uncertain environment have direct impact on the life or death of another person. Healthcare professionals take this responsibility very seriously. The need to "not make a mistake" in a sea of uncertain outcomes places pressures on members of IHTs that are different from those placed on members of most SDWTs.

There are additional differences between IHTs and SDWTs. SDWTs in business settings appear to focus more on teaching skills that promote interaction with the broader organization.[8] Because of their interests in continuous improvement, SDWTs also promote learning a technical base for evaluation. Thanks to IHI and TeamSTEPPS, this is changing for healthcare teams. However, sometimes the most critical elements of health care are the most difficult to accurately measure, as exemplified in the following case:

> **Cory:** "I was speaking with the head of our Quality Improvement Department. She expressed that she was very proud they had reduced the number of errors in medications being dispensed on the medical units. I asked if they had ever looked at whether the right medicines were being prescribed for each patient's situation. She said they had not."

SDWTs also excel at cross training and the learning of self-management techniques by all team members. On the other hand, IHTs have better addressed issues related to interprofessional differences. Although health care does not attempt to cross-train health providers, in the past 20 years there has been an acceptance of lesser-trained healthcare providers doing work for which more highly trained providers used to be exclusively responsible. IHTs also help team members recognize and capitalize on areas of skill overlap. Rather than focusing on time-consuming management skills, IHTs address functional/shared leadership and help members assume appropriate leadership roles.[9]

Similarities

Despite the differences between IHTs and business teams, there are also many similarities. During the 1980s and 1990s, a newer sector of health care was developing its own concept of teams. Healthcare managers increasingly emerged from the business community and schools of healthcare management. These individuals had been trained in the business model of teamwork. Although they were taught to believe in teams, they held different images of "team" from those held by health professionals.

Continual Existence of Entering and Leaving Members

The continual existence of entering and leaving members is a problem for both IHTs and SDWTs in business. IHTs seldom choose their members, and it is common for members to terminate and new members to join. The structure of healthcare systems encourages high staff turnover and rotating key disciplines like nursing. Healthcare administrators may borrow staff from one specialized team to cover shortages in another specialized team. SDWTs cover these inevitabilities by cross-training. In health care, coverage is just expected. Like SDWTs in business settings, IHTs are subject to downsizing. Frequent reframing of organizational priorities often results in changes in external funding for health care and a hesitancy to pay for primary patient support services by disciplines such as social work, dietetics, or occupational therapy. Urgent patient care tasks and the lack of time for team development activities in health settings prohibit the entire IHT from meeting the needs of each new member. And, finally, although SDWTs talk about team development, like IHTs they often don't take the time to meet the needs of new members.

Bilevel or Incongruous Development

As a result of changing personal, professional, and team issues— including moderate to high membership turnover—an IHT and a SDWT have at least two developmental levels: (1) the level of the team, and (2) the level of the individual member. Lacoursiere[10] concluded that, in a group, isolated individuals *can* reflect phases differing from the group's developmental phase. Based on our discussions with members of a variety of IHTs and SDWTs, it appears common for individual members to reflect different phases of development from the team as a whole. It is expected that new IHT members will be at different developmental phases from the rest of the IHT. Also, ongoing members may regress to earlier phases or simply not move as rapidly through the phases as other members.

As their worlds merge, professionals trained in health care may become more like those trained in business, and many IHTs are already reflecting that transition. The issues healthcare professionals must ponder include how far into the world of business they are willing to travel; how adoption of business terminology changes their values; where the line is between caring and cost efficiency; and what are the ethical implications for patient care. During the past 16 years, as the business of health care has grown, it has teamed with nonprofit entities like IHI and governmental organizations like the AHRQ. These entities have worked together to place evaluation, safety, and quality improvement at the forefront of teamwork. It remains to be seen if what emerges will be the type of team that can both manage itself and address the complex problems of patients.

Summary

This chapter has provided a working definition of an IHT that can serve as the basis for discussion and evaluation of other team definitions. It has also provided a comparison between some of the characteristics of healthcare teams and those of business teams. In discussing IHTs with others, having the "one true definition" is not as important as agreeing on a definition in order to achieve common ground and start working together. This chapter outlined many of the variables inherent in IHTs and SDWTs. Hopefully, it will prompt you to ask questions when team definitions are assumed and not made explicit. Sharing our definitions is the first step in promoting true dialogue about IHTs. Through this dialogue, healthcare providers will establish a foundation from which to advance the science of IHTs and create functional models for training, practice, and research.

Despite, or perhaps because of, the heightened interest in making health care a profitable enterprise, the lure of interprofessional health care grows, especially in the expanding areas of outpatient care, chronic care, and community health care. Increasingly, health professionals know that they cannot provide good care for all patients through autonomous practice. Business leaders in health care realize they need to address the needs of patients with complex and chronic problems that lead to repeat hospitalizations. As the renewed interest in interprofessional healthcare teamwork gains steam, there are many questions about the new partnerships between those trained in health care vs. business models. Hopefully, these new initiatives will propel us forward and keep us from repeating the mistakes of our collective past.

Questions for Discussion

1. As a healthcare professional, what kinds of barriers to efficiency and effectiveness, if any, have you encountered from the management side of your organization?

2. As a business or management professional, what kinds of barriers to efficiency or effectiveness, if any, have you encountered from healthcare professionals?

3. What are some ways you have found to overcome differences in values between healthcare and business professionals?

4. Have you noticed differences between teams that you have worked on? To what would you attribute those differences?

4

Communication in an Interprofessional Team Environment: Narratives, Myths, Metaphors, and Mental Images[*]

A Story

The young medical resident responded to a call for help from the nurses on the ward caring for an elderly man who had been admitted to the hospital. He had become increasingly agitated and difficult to manage, especially at night. He kept getting up at 2:00 a.m. and insisting that he had to get dressed and go to work. No amount of explanation from the staff that he was now in the hospital and did not have to get up seemed to be effective, so the nurses asked the resident to provide a chemical restraint that would reduce the difficult behaviors and make the patient more manageable.

The resident complied with the nurses' request and ordered the medication. Unfortunately, however, the patient had a significant reaction to it

---

* Parts of this chapter are based on two previous publications: Clark, P. G. (2014). Narrative in interprofessional education and practice: Implications for professional identity, communication, and teamwork. *Journal of Interprofessional Care, 28*: 34–39; and Clark, P. G. (2015). Emerging themes in the use of narrative in geriatric care: Implications for patient-centered practice and interprofessional teamwork. *Journal of Aging Studies, 34*: 177–182.

and died the next day. Only later did the staff learn that the elderly patient had been a milkman all his life, and he had to get up every morning at 2:00 a.m. to go to his job for the local dairy company. Had they known this man's story, they would have handled his apparently difficult behavior differently by reassuring him that someone else had taken his milk route while he was in the hospital and that his job would be there for him when he returned.

The devastated resident decided that he would use this incident at every opportunity to share with his fellow healthcare providers the importance of learning about the backgrounds of their patients and using this information to provide effective, sensitive, and personal care that recognized the "person behind the patient." In addition, the resident realized that he needed to communicate more effectively with other providers, such as nurses and social workers, to learn more from them about the patient's life and background.

Introduction

Poor communication among healthcare professionals is the leading root cause of sentinel events in hospitals.[1] In reality, lack of communication, miscommunication, and ineffective communication are common problems in all areas of health care. The Houghton Mifflin Dictionary defines communication as "the exchange of thoughts, messages, or information, as by speech, signals, writing, or behavior."[2] When we apply this definition to interprofessional healthcare teams (IHTs), the possibilities for communication problems become multiplied by the number of individuals within the IHT, their patients and caregivers, and members of other teams. Indeed, a major reason for allocating time to develop and maintain an IHT is to reduce the possibilities for miscommunication.

Each team member comes to the IHT with ideas and assumptions about what a team should be like, how its members should behave and relate to the patient, and how they should communicate with each other. Based on our previous education, socialization, and experience, we all carry in our heads different narratives, metaphors, myths, or idealized conceptions for how teams should work. These images and stories are largely based on our professional identities, learned ways of relating to the patient rooted in our professional education, and our (perhaps naïve) beliefs about what a team should be and how it should work.

Members of different professions develop preferences for how to identify and solve problems as part of their education and socialization into their profession. Although differences in problem-solving and communication do occur between individuals from the same discipline, they appear to be more common between different disciplines. Communication preferences may also differ along generational lines and between different specialties within health care. This is especially the case with the advent and expansion of digital and electronic methods for communication. IHTs can use insights into all these differences as tools to improve communication and team functioning. Thus, communication is an essential skill for team members to acquire, both in its own right and for its effect on how the team works together to improve patient care and outcomes.

Understanding communication challenges in healthcare settings requires knowledge of three dimensions that focus on different levels of relationships: (1) *relationship to oneself*, in which education and socialization in the development of one's own professional identity, values, and "voice" shape one's approach to communication, (2) *relationship to the patient*, in which one's unique profession's approach influences patterns of communication with the patient and the family, and (3) *relationship to the IHT*, in which communication involves the challenges of contributing one's own voice to the emerging dialogue of the team as a whole. These three layers of communication are related and provide a structure for conceptualizing communication as a set of interrelated behaviors. Throughout this discussion, we will draw on the different dimensions of language and narrative, including the concepts of stories, jargon, myths, and mental images.

Professional Identity: Relationship to Oneself

Donald Schön's[3] work on educating the reflective practitioner serves as the starting point for our thinking about how one's development as a healthcare professional is the foundation for communication in IHTs. The reflective practitioner is one who has mastered the dual bases of what it means to be a professional: (1) the scientific foundation of a profession, which includes the technical knowledge and skills required for competency, and (2) the artistic elements, which are related to navigating the complex, complicated, and uncharted areas of professional practice that are the domain of moral ambiguity, value conflict, and ethical dilemmas. As noted elsewhere in this book (Chapter 10), these two dimensions of professional practice can be linked to the cognitive and normative maps that characterize a profession. The former constitutes the epistemological foundation of a profession—its ability to gather, analyze, and utilize information; the latter is related to the ontological basis—what it means to be a particular profession, based on values that underpin professional identity.

Relevant to IHTs, the ontological dimension of professional practice is expressed as a part of identity and is embodied in narrative methods and skills. "Professional narratives are highly specialized forms of narrative that draw on the expertise and expert knowledge that professionals bring to their work."[4] They lead to a recognition of the limits of one's own knowledge and the need for contributions from other professions to create a complete picture of the patient's story. Professionals need to step back from their own situational perspectives to identify and incorporate others' points of view. This process has been termed "perspective transformation," or "decentering," and is discussed at more length in Chapter 10. This ability is key to promoting effective communication on the IHT.

It hardly seems surprising to say that every IHT is built from the various core healthcare disciplines that make it up. However, this apparently simple statement belies an important fact: It is the differences among these professions that need to be recognized and addressed if we are to promote effective communication that both celebrates and bridges them. Research has characterized different health and social care professions as representing differing cultures or subcultures. It is this variety of thought and language, standards of appearance and behavior, and such factors as personal and professional identity that are shaped by professional socialization and education.[5] In particular, it is the different sets of values characterizing differing health professionals that create perceptions of the patient and each other that make communication on IHTs such a challenge.[6,7]

Indeed, it is these different underlying values that are the foundation of professional narratives, which are the "professional scripts"[8] and the "stories to live by"[9] of health and social care providers. Professionals literally see the world differently through the lenses created by these differing values.[10] In keeping with this description, Walker[11] refers to this as a narrative of moral identity, revealing what one values, cares about, and responds to. This concept is akin to the idea discussed earlier, based on the work of Schön, of the artistic or ontological dimensions of professional practice. Seeing the world differently also means that varying providers frame the patient's problems in different ways, revealing a separate set of solutions to those problems. Narrative analysis of these differences reveals differing literary genres[12] that are developed to reflect certain standards and structures for their development as case presentations and their use in clinical settings. "Every profession has distinctive expectations about how professional stories must be told, ranging from the layout and sequence of the arguments to the style of the sentence structure used."[13]

For example, health and social care professions may have either a more biomedical or a more psychosocial perspective that determines their communication styles[14, 15] For physicians, "the technical world of medicine uses a speech genre . . . that does not lend itself well to a full exploration of contextual issues,"[16] such as everyday social relationships and activities.

In contrast, social work emphasizes these psychosocial aspects of the patient's lifeworld, even developing an approach to care that values the accomplishments, strengths, and resources of the client—as opposed to their needs, weaknesses, and problems.[17] In addition, social workers are trained to "rule in" those factors in a patient's narrative that might be left out by other, more biomedically oriented professions.[18] Factors crucial for the development of a care plan—such as a client's work, income, family, and social network—are likely to be introduced into a social work assessment.

Provider–Patient Communication

As noted in the case study story at the beginning of this chapter, challenges with communication in healthcare settings are increasingly linked to understanding the patient as a person and to developing patient-centered care, especially in IHTs.[19] As Clarke and colleagues suggest, "Person-centered care necessitates that practitioners learn more about the . . . person as an individual, together with a better understanding of the patient's personal meanings, experiences, and attitudes."[20] Indeed, the narrative relationship between the professional and the patient is the foundation of health and social care. In this regard, we must keep in mind that different professions use differing narrative methods and structures to cocreate the patient's story.

Different professions see things differently, even when they look at the same patient, because the epistemological and ontological foundations of their professions are different. Information made available to the provider is selectively processed, packaged, and presented by different professionals within the framework developed by their education and socialization as a professional. These worldviews may be more biomedical or more psychosocial in orientation, more acute or more chronic in focus, and more disease-based or functional in nature. This fact may set up an IHT for conflicts around assessment approaches, focus of professional efforts, locus of responsibility, and the pace of clinical action.[21] In addition, different professions may define the patient's problems differently, thereby setting up a range of conflicting solutions to them and dissimilar narrative genres in the process.[22]

The essence of the narrative approach to communication draws attention to the importance of having the patient's voice at the center of what health and social care should be all about. Walker[23] describes the dynamic between the provider and the patient as a narrative of relationship, in which the story is jointly constructed, interpreted, and modified in an ongoing, dynamic interaction between the two interlocutors. This relationship has two dimensions: temporal and integrative. Over time—past, present, and future—both the provider and the patient jointly construct the patient narrative, incorporating perspectives from both participants.

Importantly, the voices of both participants must be balanced in this communicative relationship. If one or the other version of the story dominates, there may be distortion in the story, with domination by one voice over the other. For example, the format of the "proper" medical narrative may reflect the technical–scientific world of the physician taking priority over the actual life experience of the patient. In addition, a patient narrative may be "abbreviated or distorted in clinical applications as practitioners have sought to fit rich and varied narratives into the format of the 'admissions form' or 'clinical history.'"[24] A similar outcome may occur when a traditional method of assessment focuses more on the patient's deficits or deficiencies than his or her strengths and resources.[25]

For example, different health and social care professionals may approach various types of patients (such as older adults) with "master narratives" that are generalized or archetypal formats for thinking about a patient, his or her problems, and the set of solutions to be considered in addressing them. Such "stock plots" or "character types" can simplify the work of the health or social care professional by providing "off the shelf" prepackaged short-cuts to a patient assessment. The danger, however, is that such a simplified approach will ignore unique contextual or particularistic factors by seeing only the more universal or paradigmatic ones.

For example, in geriatrics the "stock plot" of a narrative of decline for older adults may lead to ageism and discrimination toward the older patient and result in low-quality care. In such a situation, "counter stories" that question such a discriminatory picture may need to be presented. As Nelson[26] suggests, the older adult "who is caught in a narrative of decline . . . needs a counter story that allows her to sustain or retain a practical identity that is threatened by something or someone she can't control." Finally, the nature of conditions presented by patients that serve as the basis for their narratives is also evolving, with implications for the development of narratives co-constructed by provider and patient. The nature and work of health and social care providers will change as chronic diseases and multiple comorbidities become more prevalent. In such situations, the importance of quality of life, and not simply its length, will increase, with a corresponding emphasis on the patient's values and wishes and the associated goals of care. Thus, narrative approaches to communication will become increasingly important in inviting the patient's perspective in the development of the clinical narrative, which will become less about solving acute problems and more about managing chronic ones.

Communication among Healthcare Professionals

Understanding communication among members of an IHT involves examining different dimensions of the use of words and stories by team members: (1) narratives, (2) words and their meanings, (3) business jargon, and (4) unspoken influences on team communication.

Narratives

As mentioned earlier, the use of patient narratives underlies effective communication among the members of an IHT. The sharing of different narratives, based on differing professional genres, becomes the foundation for developing an integrated patient assessment and care plan. In this sense, members of an IHT become members of an interprofessional "narrative community of practice" in which the presentation of different clinical narratives results in a multivocal "layering" of the story line as each team member presents his or her own unique version of the patient's story. Interestingly, it is this exchange among members of the team that can actually sharpen each profession's own sense of identity and uniqueness, as they experience the diversity in the ways in which professionals see, hear, and experience the patient's story as coauthored through the lens of their own background, training, and socialization.

We now focus on the interaction among the different health and social care professions on the IHT and their integration of assessment information and its use in developing a unified care plan. If each narrative represented by a profession on the team embodies a unique, if incomplete, picture of the patient's story, then it is essential that they come together to construct a complete picture of the patient. It is the dialogue and discourse among the members of the IHT that literally "assembles" the patient in his or her entirety. This reminds us of a colleague who had a fantasy in which he would have a dinner party and invite all the health professionals who took care of different "parts" of him, so they could literally assemble him around the table as a complete patient. The limits of each profession's expertise and knowledge create "interpretive gaps" in the narrative, spaces that must be filled in by the differing perspectives and contributions of different professions. For example, Hsu and McCormack[27] discuss how the reinterpretation, reconfiguration, and reintegration of different provider narratives are necessary to construct a holistic picture of the patient.

This need for many clinical voices to be raised in the creation of the patient's narrative has been termed "dialogism" in teamwork, which requires that the participants in the narrative exchange go beyond simply hearing the information to reflecting on its significance and how it is related to all the data being presented by the different team members.[28] This "multivocality" of teamwork may depend on the creation of "microcommunities . . . as the venues for communication about our beliefs, values, preferences, [and] narratives."[29]

The achievement of true multivocality by a team is the key to its achieving the kind of integrated communication required for effective collaboration, and it can enhance team cohesion[30] and lead to improved team effectiveness and patient outcomes. For example, McClelland and Sands[31] found that the absence of a team member who possessed a critical piece of information about the patient had a negative effect on patient care. Similarly, Opie[32] argues that how differing representations are made by different team members has a powerful effect on the team's options for action.

In this context, it is interesting to note that narrative training for interprofessional teams improves team cohesiveness and function, leading to a greater ability to provide high-quality patient care[33] and enhance insight by team members into the backgrounds of others.[34] The presentation and discussion of patient narratives has also been shown to positively affect the understanding of where one's own professional identity falls along the continuum of discourse about patient care as well as lead to an increased appreciation for the perspectives of others on the team.[35]

Words and Their Meanings

Professionals in healthcare settings also frequently use jargon as a short cut when communicating with a colleague. Although the terminology used by professionals from one discipline can be confusing to professionals from other fields, it often goes unquestioned. Websites for various medical teaching facilities list common medical catchphrases with their abbreviations. Each discipline has its own set of jargon, catchphrases, and abbreviations that also vary in different parts of the country and throughout the world.

For example, Rice University[36] has a compendium of medical jargon consisting of over 800 words, some of which have more than one meaning. Medical acronyms also vary between different parts of the world and throughout the United States. Nurses might use slang like PITA ("pain in the ass"), CAH ("crazy as hell"), and FMPS ("fluff my pillow syndrome")[37] in communicating with other nurses, and frequently use acronyms in verbal communication and charting.[38] Social workers tend to use jargon like *holistic, process, intervention, entitlement, advocacy, empower, build rapport,* and *engage,*[39] and acronyms like "AODA (alcohol and other drug abuse); MOW (meals on wheels); and IL (independent living)"[40] for services they frequently use for patients. Nurses and social workers overlap in their values and philosophies of care, and both professions use jargon related to a systems approach to care that has slightly different meanings.

A search of the Internet reveals that jargon relative to health care is discussed in many posts from the United Kingdom but few from the United States. Some authors who have reviewed the use of jargon think it is an exclusionary force, a way of segregating a group and allowing them to feel superior to others who aren't in the group. Other authors believe jargon and acronyms are a uniting force in that their use helps bind a group together, making members feel a part of a whole. The way words are used can define a culture, as discussed previously, and that is a reason why different disciplines develop their own languages. As a member of an IHT, it is important that you be tuned into the heavy use of jargon and question terms you don't understand. Questioning jargon can uncover discrepancies that prevent a common understanding of a complex problem. One of the benefits of having well-developed IHTs is that members feel comfortable questioning each other's procedures, decisions, and jargon.

Business Jargon

Professionals in business settings have their own set of jargon and catchphrases such as "actionable, best practices, buy-in, close the loop, critical path, dialogue, and functionality"[41] that emerged from a culture far removed from health care but are increasingly being used in healthcare settings. The field of business is known for using jargon and catchphrases in its marketing and training approaches to products and services. One article suggests much of the jargon used in business like *strategic, blocking, ballpark figure*, and *end run*, relates to war and sports.[42] The author expresses concern that the "macho language" commonly used in business goes against the real mission of business that is supposed to be helping people. Some might argue about the real mission of business, but few would openly argue that helping people should be the real mission of health care.

Despite the professed mission of health care to help people, one of the most widely adopted healthcare team training programs in the United States uses war and sports terminology in its curriculum. In its online master trainer course, the Agency for Healthcare Research and Quality (AHRQ) outlines tools and strategies that move healthcare teams from barriers to outcomes. Words, phrases, and acronyms used by the Team-STEPPS Model include: *Hand off, Call-Out, IPASSTHEBATON, Time Out, Brief, Huddle, Debrief, Two Challenge Rule, STEP*, and *CUS*.[43]

In the past 20 years, healthcare professionals have also been expected to learn and use business terms centered on quality improvement terminology that emerged from manufacturing. Healthcare professionals felt compelled to adopt this terminology. It is easy to envision fast evolving healthcare systems where healthcare professionals do not have the time to develop trust between team members. Chances are very high that they would not feel comfortable questioning the jargon used by other professionals, including business professionals, if they felt they did not understand it. Or, perhaps in their rush to provide health care, professionals assume there is a common understanding when there is not.

Health care has become a product within the business model, establishing a race to control costs and raise money for investors. Business jargon like *working to the top of your license, coaching, core competency, brand, best practice, stakeholders*, and *value-added* have been introduced into the healthcare providers' lexicon. And healthcare providers have willingly adopted acronyms like *B2B, B2C, COO, CFO, CEO, KPO*, and *ROI* as part of their repertoire. As healthcare managers increasingly apply pressure to use statistics in forming and refining approaches to care, providers have seemingly accepted the business model as part of their practice. Perhaps the use of business jargon makes healthcare providers feel an equal part of the management sphere of influence.

Unspoken Influences on Team Communication

Members of IHTs also harbor images of the teams (past and present) on which they have served. Negative and positive experiences are remembered at both conscious and subconscious levels and undoubtedly affect how members either communicate or don't communicate with team-mates. Images of teams are also a reflection of interpersonal experiences that team members have had. These interpersonal experiences with family, friends, and acquaintances lay the groundwork for the way healthcare providers view themselves in relation to a team and for how quickly they assimilate into the team. The team proficiencies in which health providers engage as part of their training and work experience can be expressed in metaphors, myths, and mental images.

Metaphors

Metaphors represent figurative languages that we all develop based on our life experiences.[44] Healthcare professionals grew up, either as observers or as participants, with varied team experiences: softball, volleyball, spelling, and debate teams. These team experiences plus our life experiences in our families and other more formal groups have etched metaphors of teams in our minds. Metaphors that health professionals collect during primary professional training may be altered once those individuals leave their training. Also, the metaphors continue to change, based on the experiences that practitioners encounter in their work. Although sports team metaphors are those to which we have most often been exposed, they might not be the predominant team metaphors for healthcare professionals.

In the not-too-distant past, the metaphors healthcare providers preferred were not those from sports, war, or the business model. Drinka and Miller[45] studied several groups of healthcare providers to ascertain their metaphors related to IHTs. The research revealed that health professionals who worked on teams generally applied more nonsports than sports metaphors to teamwork (e.g., music, learning, synergistic effects, and the weather). When team members did apply sports metaphors to teams (after being prompted), they often had differing interpretations of a particular sports metaphor. For example, the sports metaphor of football was seen by one team member as "teamwork with good coaches" and by another as "a bunch of unfriendly quarterbacks—too many directors—too few doers."

Study respondents also reported using different metaphors in current practice from those they had used at the end of their formal professional training. One member noted that at the culmination of his training, his metaphor for team was "figure skating—all beauty, graceful and smooth with a few falls now and then, little did I know!" After several years of practice this team member had changed his metaphor to, "a hockey team—there are fights within a team and between teams. There can be bruises (ego and physical) and disagreements, etc. but in the end it's team effort that wins." The diverse metaphors demonstrated that this individual, during his training, had a simplistic metaphor of team. However, his view of "team" matured with his practice experience as evidenced by his posttraining metaphor. Although some might interpret this individual's later metaphor as negative, it reflected the complex nature of an IHT.

Observing the way team members use metaphors can be a valuable tool in diagnosing the state of a team. When team members apply unidimensional metaphors to dynamic and complex processes, it is a clear sign that something is not working. Using unidimensional metaphors, like "a lovely flower in bloom," may indicate that either the team member is not integrated into the team or that the team is not well developed. When a unidimensional metaphor is negative, as "the patient is the puck," it might suggest unresolved team conflict. Like the team member who changed from a figure skating to a hockey metaphor, the metaphors of team members should grow dimensionally as the team itself develops.

Team members can be taught to be aware of the metaphors that they and other team members carry and to use them as a measure of the team's developmental process. It is important for an IHT to attain a common understanding of metaphors that are applied to the team by making them explicit and discussing their meanings. As a team process exercise, a team member might ask all team members to list their metaphors for the team. This could be done anonymously or as an open collective. It would be essential to discuss what the metaphors mean, whether or not a team likes their metaphors, and how the team would like to see them change over time.

Myths

Myths and legends are narratives that arise in the course of a team's development. Myths unmask the "world view" of the team's members or of the team as a whole. Myths and legends are another powerful force that teams can use in communication to develop and sustain a particular culture. One of the reasons myths are so powerful is that they tap into stories that were presented to us as children. One myth involves a powerful figure that has the capacity to save people from distress.

For example, one IHT had been struggling for a year to develop its clinical base. In the course of that development it had a formal leader who did not establish a firm direction for the team. The team was just beginning to develop its informal leadership roles. Suddenly a powerful physician was hired to be the team's director at a time when the team's funding was in jeopardy. This physician was able to reestablish the funding and evolved as the team's protector. The team members referred to him as "big daddy," and whenever members needed something they would go to him, knowing that their concerns would be heard.

Another IHT was assigned a director who was a powerful physician in the larger organization and was feared by many members of the team. One day two team members were walking down the hospital corridor and passed the team director who was speaking to a group of students. He bellowed down the hall at them, "Don't you stop and say hello to god?" Although it was the director's way of making a joke, it was clear that he saw himself as powerful. Because many team members did not feel free to approach this director, they often let team business slide. Communication between team members decreased. Team conflicts that should have been addressed were ignored and the team began to collapse.

Perhaps a team has struggled collectively against a system that had little faith in the team's ability to manage a particular type of patient. If the healthcare team proves successful at providing good care to those patients who were deemed unsalvageable by the system, a myth might develop about that team. That team might also see itself as able to perform superhuman feats. One healthcare team saw itself as a low-flying plane, able to evade the radar of bureaucratic rules that the organization imposed to keep change from occurring. Within the system the team was seen as a maverick, not accepted by most but secretly admired and envied. As one member of the team observed:

Carmen: "I am a case manager for a group of IHTs. One IHT harbored a myth of limitless creativity. The team was sure that it could solve any complex problem that came its way. It was caring for a particularly difficult 90-year-old patient who had been a prominent member of our small community. The patient had diabetes, dementia, congestive heart failure, and multiple other problems. He was demanding of constant attention from his family caregivers and was wearing them out. The team was expending inordinate amounts of energy and resources on their communications to find ways to keep the patient and family satisfied. The patient's son became very frustrated at the effect his father's constant care had on his mother. At a particularly frustrating time, he asked a team member if they couldn't just give his father a pill to make him better. Rather than realizing their limits, the team began struggling even harder to find a solution to this situation. During a team meeting, members were re-examining the patient's medications and questioning once again their approach when one of the team members threw a foot long plastic pill on the table. The team members burst out laughing as they realized that they were beyond realistic limits of patient care. For the moment the myth of invincibility was exploded, but I realized it would take ongoing conversation about boundary issues and the limits of our team's ability to deliver care."

Mental Images of the Team

The pictures of a team that members have in their collective unconscious can also provide an understanding of how members are communicating. An exercise we have performed during team training sessions often provides a valuable tool for examining a team's communication patterns. We ask team members individually to draw a picture of *a* team. We intentionally don't ask them to draw an image of *their* team, but they frequently do. The picture then provides a starting point for a discussion of communication patterns. A team's collective pictures can indicate the extent of the team members' experience and understanding of teams in general and of their team in particular.

Although the pictures are lines on a page, the shape and connectivity of the lines reveal a narrative and tell a story. For example, one team member might draw a fully formed circle, while another member of that same team might draw a circle consisting of disconnected lines. The different images form the impetus for a discussion. Another picture might portray some team members on one side of a fence and other team members on the other side, leading to a discussion of difficulties in communication.

Some pictures that team members draw will be detailed and others very simple. Some pictures may seem mundane, but each is a vivid indicator of team function. Many of the pictures team members draw are noteworthy. If each member of a team draws their team as a group of superheroes, it can lead to a discussion of reforming communication patterns so no team member has to bear the burden of being superhuman. Whatever form the drawings take, they are useful tools for either newly formed teams or ongoing teams to reveal and review their interactional patterns.

The important thing to note about mental images or pictures is that they often exist as implicit communication and remain unquestioned. Over time they become reified and part of a team's culture. Sometimes these images are positive and help the team develop and meet its goals. However, these images can also be destructive to the team's development and may impede team growth. Taking time to make a team's images explicit is a good team development exercise and can help a team see why it is headed in the direction of its mission; or, conversely, why it might have strayed off course.

Timing of Communication

Knowing when or when not to communicate with another provider is one of the most difficult things to learn as a healthcare provider. In health care the right communication at the right time can be critical. There can also be either too much or not enough communication. Ill-timed communication between providers can cause conflict within an IHT. For example, a nurse might initiate conflict with a physician if the physician perceives the nurse's communication as unnecessary or bothersome.

Many long-term care facilities have received violations for not reporting patient falls when they occur, because they can denote a change in a patient's condition. However, a physician who receives a call from a night shift nurse for every patient fall might resent being awakened for such communications. In fact, when a patient has many chronic illnesses, it is likely not necessary to report every fall. To resolve this team conflict it would be reasonable for the team to categorize types of falls and their consequences to establish policies for reporting falls that would serve the best interests of the patients without unnecessarily disturbing the sleep of physicians.

Summary

Although it might seem odd for healthcare professionals to dwell on their narratives, jargon, metaphors, myths, and mental images, taking time to explore them can enhance team members' ability to communicate with other team members and in turn can improve their team practice. Healthcare providers quickly learn to work hard, produce, and avoid mistakes. It is difficult to break through this veneer of hard work and caring in order to communicate about a problem the team is having. Narratives, metaphors, myths, and mental images are powerful tools that can help an IHT overcome its barriers to learning and improve efficiency of practice. Understanding how IHTs might differ from other organizational team cultures can also be useful in interacting with those cultures to enhance the work of the IHT. It is important for team members from healthcare and business backgrounds to realize their differences and similarities and identify catchphrases, metaphors, myths, and images members can use from both worlds to improve necessary communication between team members.

As in any relationship, effective communication among team members is essential, yet it is often reported to be a significant challenge to improving team functioning. Taking on this challenge requires an awareness of the different levels, dimensions, and factors in communication, and how its development and refinement is an essential skill required of all IHT members. "Keeping the lines of communication open" requires constant effort and commitment, but ultimately it is one of the key ingredients of IHT success and positive impact on patient care.

Questions for Discussion

1. What are some communication challenges that you have encountered while working on interprofessional teams? List as many as you can think of.
2. What were the underlying causes of these problems, and how did you attempt to solve them?
3. Were some of these communication problems due to differences in the ways in which different professions see the world and the patient? If so, are these problems easier or more difficult for members of an IHT to resolve?
4. Current concerns about safety problems in the U.S. healthcare system seem to suggest that better, more accurate, and more complete communication of information would go a long way in addressing them. What are some of the ways this could be accomplished?
5. What are some of the mental images you hold about different healthcare disciplines and also about working on an IHT?

5

Key Elements in Team Development and Maintenance

This chapter provides a model for understanding interprofessional healthcare teams (IHTs) as the complex, dynamic, and useful entities that they are. The first section discusses the difficulty of getting healthcare professionals to reflectively look at their team. The middle three sections outline a conceptual framework that captures the necessary components and patterns of development within an IHT. The final section addresses the efficiency of interprofessional practice. This model was developed over a period of 20 years and has been tested in an ongoing IHT.[1] It explains how IHTs must develop and work in order to solve the types of problems for which they are created. In this chapter, we will see how IHTs that are well-developed can be efficient vehicles for delivering health care in a wide range of situations. Finally, this chapter reminds us that IHTs differ from other types of teams and must be recognized as the distinct entities they are.

Pictures Are Worth a Thousand Words

It is common for healthcare professionals to view teamwork as hand-offs between members of different professions. It is no surprise, because that is the way most of us were taught to practice. During team building and team maintenance workshops, I often ask each member of the audience to individually draw a picture of a healthcare team. One of the most frequent images team members draw is a large fire burning brightly on one end of the page. On the opposite end of the page is an equally large basin of water. Between the fire and the basin, a bucket is passed person-to-person from the water basin to the fire and back again. Inevitably when I ask the team to imagine a more efficient way to put out the fire, at least one or two members of the audience suggest that everyone in the line pick up the basin in unison and pour it on the fire. Too often healthcare providers are still learning the single bucket approach to suppressing fires in health care.

While collectively pouring all the water on a fire might be the best solution for that particular fire, the question arises whether it is the right solution for all of the team's fires. The collective act of pouring water on a fire says nothing of:

- Why or how the fire was created;
- Similar fires that preceded this fire;
- How quickly the team arrived at the fire;
- Whose actions precipitated this fire;
- Which members of the team were available to extinguish the fire;
- Whether the fire could have been prevented;
- How much damage the fire caused;
- How you resolve conflicts over whose fire gets extinguished first;
- Who will clean up after the fire;
- What other leadership roles must be assumed;
- How future fires could be treated or controlled;
- How to train team members in optimum ways to extinguish and/or avoid a fire;
- How to train team members to address these issues;
- How money in the budget plays a role in such training; or
- How to negotiate training and other resources with funders and administrators.

Even when healthcare professionals are exposed to team training, it might not be sufficient to propel them to form a well-developed interprofessional team that can address a never-ending presentation of complex and unique problems.

Another frequent occurrence in team development workshops was when members of one team all drew pictures that gave glowing accounts of teamwork. Members of an IHT that was in crisis would draw pictures of flowers in bloom, people holding hands around a circle, smiling faces of team members and patients, and other positive images. Collectively these pictures were not an accurate reflection of their team. They were not even a realistic impression of a well-functioning team. They raised an index of suspicion that the team members were unable to accurately view their team or were covering up normal conflicts that occur as part of teamwork. These rosy-hued perceptions might also have been a reflection of the way their organization viewed the world.

When I couldn't seem to elicit accurate drawings of their teams, I would ask members to individually draw a picture of team conflict. Some were unable to do so. However, when prompted, most were able to picture at least one of the problems that regularly occurred on their team. Some of the more common depictions were of team members sitting around a table with ghosts in the background, team members playing tug-of-war using a large rope, team members with their backs turned while a team member was talking, team members climbing large mountains with many hazards, and one team member (frequently a nurse) pulling a cart full of other team members. When several team members depicted the same conflict, it provided a golden moment that opened up honest team communication, allowing the team to progress in its development.

Helping a team create an image for how their IHT should or does function is just a beginning. Developing and maintaining the performance of an IHT is the real challenge. The primary care clinic team described in Chapter 2 was facing patient and caregiver problems that were complex, interrelated, and indefinite. Patient problems were confounded with problems created by the larger healthcare system. Because of its place in the larger system, the team described in 2016 appeared to have less practice autonomy than the team described in 2000. Multifaceted problems, like addressing the needs of an ill caregiver when those needs conflict with the needs of an ill spouse and the economic mandates of an ever-changing healthcare system, require complex and interrelated solutions that demand well-functioning IHTs.

Four Essential Team Components and Their Variables

An understanding of the dynamics of IHTs does not come naturally for most of us. One review of team research noted that team training in the process area has little effect on improving outcomes but focusing on goals does.[2] In our experience, an IHT can focus on its goals, but unless it is also aware of its dynamics, the team's long-term outcomes will be adversely affected.

An IHT is made up of essential components that should work together to achieve the team's goals in an effective and efficient manner. Understanding how a team's components and their variables are working together is complex, and this makes it difficult to diagnose team function and dysfunction.

The organization and the team share responsibility for assuring that individual and professional practice components are in place and appropriate for the team's work. The team has internal cultural components that it cultivates through goal setting, problem solving, and conflict management. These require the team to establish appropriate structure and process. The broader organization works with the team to provide the resources to accomplish the team's mission and to keep it aligned with the mission of the organization. Finally, the team maintains itself in a growth pattern through learning, leadership, and teaching. These four components are necessary for an IHT to thrive. However, some components may be neglected, which can lead to problems in the team's ability to develop effectively into a mature entity that can withstand continuous change. The variables encompassed by these components are everchanging and interacting. The components of an IHT form the base of the team development model. Understanding these components (Table 5.1) will help team members determine where the problems lie when a team is malfunctioning.

Practice Components: Personal and Professional

Although personal characteristics are downplayed, they perform a major role during the initial formation of an IHT or following significant changes in focus or membership. The ongoing impact of personal factors on a team's members is unique to each team, and although personal characteristics such as charisma may not be a significant source of power in an existing IHT, they do affect a team's function.[3] The greatest impact of personal characteristics might be when new members enter an IHT that is already developed. In this situation, the personal factors of age, gender, cultural background, styles of relating, and charisma of members are the magnet that attracts a new member to an existing member. This attraction may be an important factor in the type of orientation a new member receives. The results will depend on which phase of team development the ongoing member is in, whether the team is in a different phase of development, and the attitude of the orienting member toward the team.

Table 5.1 The Interprofessional Healthcare Team: Components and Variables

I. Issues That Directly Influence Practice

Personal	Professional
• appreciate age/gender/culture	• become expert in your specialty
• acquire communication skills	• clarify professional values
• exhibit energy for teamwork	• respect professional differences
• understand your styles of relating	• broadly know health care
• be willing to risk/be flexible	• willingly share client
• know your leadership styles	• attain professional maturity
• remain open to new knowledge	• know roles of others
• know and understand yourself	• know systems
• respect yourself	• know how different professionals problem solve
• monitor your personal conflict styles	• allow time to work with a team
	• know when and how to work as a team

II. Intrateam Issues

Team Structure	Team Process
• establish formal leadership	• negotiate informal leadership
• recognize norms	• set goals
• determine team composition	• appreciate different values
• communicate formal professional roles	• negotiate team roles
• recognize team culture	• build trust
• recognize professional status	• communicate
• establish equal status for problem solving	• collectively define complex problems
• structure for efficient interaction	• continually problem solve/influence
• structure for innovation	• recognize and manage conflict as it arises

III. Organizational Issues

Internal Organization	External Organization
• monitor and support team's philosophy	• promote national policy that helps the team work
• allocate resources to support the team	• monitor and encourage funding sources
• establish and support flexible rules	• exhibit supportive philosophy
• simplify structure	• understand interprofessional principles

(*Continued*)

Table 5.1 (*Continued*)

IV. Actions Necessary for Team Maintenance over Time

Team	Organization
• establish time to create structure and work on process • members use power for decision making • all commit to freedom of dissent • team evaluates and manages itself • members promptly address and resolve conflict • ongoing members teach leadership to new members	• communicate organization's mission to the team • protect the team from outside negative forces • respond in a problem-solving manner to the team's requests for help • communicate organization's mission to the team • use team feedback to revise team mission • allow the team to manage itself • give constructive feedback to the team • assign sufficient time to work with a team • collect long-term data

In addition to knowledge of their own profession, professionals on an IHT should have an understanding of the knowledge and roles of other team members. This understanding develops interprofessional trust and a willingness to share clients. Although the collective expertise of the practitioners on an IHT should address the complex needs of patients, the planned structuring of this collective expertise is very difficult. Unlike therapy, encounter, and task groups, where membership can be carefully planned, IHT membership is subject to shifts in organizational priorities, often the result of changes or cutbacks in external funding. An IHT's membership is also affected by two phenomena that are common in health settings, that is, a high rate of staff turnover and the practice of rotating staff.[4]

Professionals within any profession differ in their level of knowledge and in their professional maturity. At times the membership of an IHT might not reflect any well-conceived plan, and the combined knowledge of the professionals assigned could be insufficient to meet either the team or patient needs. It is therefore important for a team to periodically monitor its personal and professional expertise and to match them to the needs of the patients who are served by the team. Continuing professional education should be a constant. This is also one reason a team must maintain strong ties to administration, so adjustments in staffing and education can be made when necessary.

Intrateam Components: Structure and Process

Initial team development and continued team training are part of the team's internal structure and process. Developing and maintaining the intrateam components of the IHT can help members understand differences in individual and professional characteristics, and ultimately should improve the team's output. Intrateam components reflect both the needs of its patients and the survival needs of the team. The issue of trust is central to the development of the team. It involves knowledge of role performance (i.e., consistency of action). "I trust you because I know that you will do what you are supposed to do." The affective component of trust involves emotional bonds between members. These are based on developing a consistency of action that involves structures and processes.

Establishing the internal structure of the team is one of the first tasks for a new team. Internal structure might include team mission, goals, protocols for patient care, what kinds of meetings will be held, who will formally lead, expected roles, and what mechanisms will be used for informal communication. Health professionals have a love–hate relationship with meetings. Some think of them as the bane of their existence, and others think of them as necessary. Formal meetings are only one tool for communication and sharing information. Informal meetings and telephone conversations are more common and perhaps more important tools for team communication.

E-mail, voice mail, texting, and progress notes are additional means of information sharing, but they are not good forms of communication as they do not permit interactive dialogue. As part of a team's structure, policies for using these tools should be written and adapted to the needs of the team, as illustrated in the following two cases:

Tara: "I have been a nurse for thirty years and I know the way a team utilizes technology to communicate can hinder teamwork. Now we have textpaging. Instead of calling the doctor to explain what is going on, team members send a text message to the doctors on their phones. What information does that give the doctor? I was orienting a young nurse to the team. I asked what he was going to do first. I said 'Let's call the doctor.' He said 'I want to textpage.' I said 'Not with this going on. We need to call the doctor right now.' Sometimes we need to have this conversation because doctors and nurses are trained so differently. They think differently. The young nurse at the end of a day said, 'Now I know how to talk to a doctor.'"

June: "The younger professionals often take the easy way out. I would tell the nurses to put something on the list because we needed to talk to the doctor about it. I would introduce a new nurse to the medical team, and say the doctor is going to tell you about what is going on. The next day I was talking to the same nurse, and a doctor actually came and asked the nurse for information. That was a surprise to the nurse."

Team structure usually is more static than team process, and therefore is easier for new members to learn. However, even team structures must continually adapt to changes in the organizational environment. As the team develops, it should continually ensure that its structures for problem solving and recording promote team dialogue. Left to their own devices, there is a strong tendency for healthcare professionals to retreat to their discipline-specific modes for delineating, solving, and recording complex problems. When charts are sectioned by discipline, it is a good indication that the team is not interprofessional. The structure of patient treatment plans and assessment protocols can help prevent this from happening. The treatment plan should be a unified and dynamic document to which all disciplines relate. Problems should be written globally as interprofessional problems to which relevant disciplines can connect. An interprofessional problem encompasses those issues preventing a patient from achieving maximum independence. Progress notes should relate to the interprofessional treatment plan and all team members should write in the same section of the chart.

Team process and structure are interactive. For example, team process can be facilitated or hindered by strategically placing the desks of professionals from different disciplines. Placing team members' offices on different floors or in different buildings can strain efficient team communication. Structuring specific times to be on a particular unit is a formal way to enhance informal communication. New team members can be placed in close proximity to established members to both hasten and shape orientation. Team members taking an active role in program improvement can quickly alter team structure to meet the team's needs.

Establishing formal and informal leadership within the team can alter the authority roles and power structures of different professionals. A team physician may have higher authority than a nurse or social worker in terms of clinical decision making, but the nurse or social worker might be the formal team leader. Either leader can have a profound influence on how the team makes clinical decisions. A physician, social worker, nurse, or any team member will assume leadership roles, as their professional or personal skills are needed in specific situations.

A team adopts processes for accomplishing its work and over time these processes become norms, a part of the team's unwritten rules. A team's norms may include how decisions are made, leadership is carried out, and conflict is managed. Norms can address either task or socioemotional issues. Procedures and roles develop as unquestioned norms early in a team's development. Cultural norms that define a team's values and collective beliefs usually take longer to form. However, it is quite possible for several powerful team members to share cultural norms and thus speed up the assimilation of those norms into the team's work.

For example, team members who came from a teaching background might all apply the cultural norm of teaching and learning to the team. That team will develop with that norm until enough new members without that norm enter the team and overtly or covertly challenge the norm. That prompts the team to work on the process of reaffirming or changing the norm. As a team develops, its cultural norms (good and bad) gain strength and become more resistant to change. For this reason, it is good team practice for members to periodically identify and question a team's unwritten rules.

Informal and formal roles and tasks are negotiated around the team's goals. The initial goal setting and planning for patient care activities, record keeping, and administrative activities are at the heart of team decision making. New team members should be taught the informal and formal roles of team members and should be invited to openly question those roles. Ideally, team members will periodically examine the process factors that promote or hinder their interdependent problem solving.

Organizational Components: Internal and External

It is difficult for an IHT to grow without having established effective relations with its organizational environment. Unlike a task group that is structured to accomplish a specific task within a defined time period, an IHT survives over time by managing its resources within the confines of current market and political conditions. The team can strengthen its leadership position in the organization by periodically engaging in systems analysis and environmental scanning to recognize differences between its culture and the organization's culture. The rules of the broader external organization—congressional mandates or a changing mission in the CEO's office—can be applied to teams in rigid or flexible ways. It is imperative that team members interact with the administration via committee membership, informal communication, and formal administrative channels to monitor changing organizational climates. This organizational component is often left out of IHT curricula, yet it is one of the most important variables for a team's survival. When teams do not form and sustain viable and reciprocal relationships with the organization, there is a danger of developing a "we" vs. "they" attitude. If such a situation develops, the team will usually suffer.

There are many emerging organizational structures that can support IHTs. However, IHTs in healthcare organizations are often structured as matrix systems. The members of the team may be hired and have their performance appraisals written by the director of their professional department, hopefully with input from a member(s) of the team. Team members must therefore learn to strike some balance between their professional department and their IHT. The IHT generally becomes stronger when the balance is in favor of the team.

Organizations may need to intervene in situations where there is a power struggle between the team and a department head. For example, if a department head continually schedules departmental meetings during the only time that the team has to meet, the problem needs to be addressed, either by the team member from that discipline or by someone higher in the team's administrative structure. If a department head feels threatened by or somehow disrespects the team, it is critical to engage quickly with an administrator who has authority over both entities.

Problems can arise when some team members are accountable not to their respective disciplinary department, but to a supervisor who is from another discipline. If that supervisor does not have a good understanding of the disciplinary cultures of each of the team's members it can lead to misunderstandings and a potential devaluation of a specific discipline.

Components Necessary for Team Maintenance over Time

Team maintenance is the fourth major part of the IHT model, and its central focus is functional or informal leadership, not necessarily linked to any management position. Anderson and Gevitz[5] described the team approach in general hospitals as one in which no member takes on total responsibility. However, for an IHT to survive over time, every team member must assume some responsibility for team maintenance. If the IHT is a self-managing team, all of its members should be expected to assume leadership functions. This leadership may be different from the formal leadership that is part of the structural component of the team, that is, this leadership is different from the position of team manager.

Functional or informal leadership relates to the ability of each team member to take on leadership roles as team tasks call for their expertise. It is leadership that is assumed by the member of the team who is the most competent to assume it in a given situation. This concept of informal leadership refers to members' obligations to monitor and question how individual practice components, intrateam components, and broader organizational components promote the team's goals. When team members assume informal leadership, they assume power for decision making in regard to change.

To maintain its capacity for interdependent collaborative decisions and to survive over time, it is imperative that the team perform its maintenance functions. This team maintenance variable addresses the ability of all members to use power for dissent and decision making. On a developed team, each team member has power for decision making. However, each team member's power is not equal, since each member has a different body of knowledge and varied experience. Attention to this area can direct the team toward collaboration and innovation. The paradox and central assumption in this IHT model is that the team (not individual members) controls the power for its internal decision making. However, the team cannot control the power for decision making unless every member takes some responsibility for informal leadership. The assumption is that a mature IHT has developed sufficiently so that control of decision making power is not held by only one or two members, and the sense of having power for decision making is perceived by every member including support staff. A functioning IHT can take many forms and have a variable mix of professionals, but it is not well developed until it promotes the engagement of all members in interdependent collaboration.

Evolution of the Team and Its Members

The four components of IHTs and their variables not only interact with one another, but also they relate to the five phases of development and decision making: *forming, norming, confronting, performing,* and *leaving*. Each phase focuses on particular tasks and behaviors as it emphasizes different variables within the team model. Members may be in different phases from other team members, focusing on different team issues. The three main recurring phases are *norming, confronting,* and *performing*. The *forming* and *leaving* phases are in the model because they have significant, albeit intermittent, impact on a continuing IHT. Because of the urgency of the work in healthcare settings, the initial *forming* phase can be very transitional. With reference to the *leaving* phase, the entire team seldom dissolves. These two phases have more relevance to individual members who enter or leave an existing IHT, but they can also have profound effects on the team. The rate of staff turnover is an important variable in the development and maintenance of any organization. However, the reactions that continuing members have to a *leaving* member and the eventual introduction of a replacement dictate the importance of these two phases to any given team. The recurring influence of the *leaving* phase is the potential to advance or return the team to one of the other recurring phases.

The *team* phase represents the phase of the majority of members. However, it is common for individual members to perceive themselves in a developmental phase that differs from that of the collective team. New team members might influence the entire team or some of its members to revert to a less advanced phase. Also, members experiencing changes in their personal or professional lives might alter their commitment to the team and regress in relation to the *team's* phase.

Lack of staff can prompt supervisors to assign team members from other areas of the organization to the team. Often these team members are assigned to the team for low percentages of time. This limited commitment may impede a member's progression to more advanced phases of development in relation to the team. Members with less than full-time commitments to the team might have difficulty keying in to the developmental phase of the entire team. The influence that part-time and transient members have on the further development of a well-functioning team is unclear and is likely dependent on personal and professional factors that they possess.

When members leave the team, informal leadership shifts. A new member might be expected to assume a leadership role based on performance of a prior member from the same professional discipline. Assuming a key leadership role can prompt even a new member to move quickly to a more advanced phase of team development.[6] It is important for administrators and team leaders to realize that the stalled development of an IHT might be the result of limited resources to address the team's work, lack of guidance in team development, or limited time to address process or structural issues. Table 5.2 depicts the phases of IHT development and suggests some interventions to help achieve the tasks necessary to move through or maintain each phase.

Forming Phase

Members of IHTs are usually rushed to form a team and to begin performing their duties from their discipline's perspective. Instead of establishing team goals and roles or identifying personal and professional attributes that might help a team form or work through inevitable conflicts, an IHT will likely repress the conflict and charge into the *norming*

Table 5.2   **Developmental Phases of Interprofessional Healthcare Teams: Symptoms and Interventions**

Phase I: Forming

Symptoms	Interventions
Superficially share name and background information.	Create icebreakers (potlucks, informal discussions).
Members size up and test each other; categorize by professional roles and status.	Discuss formal and potential informal roles of members; verbalize stated team goals.
Members guarded, more impersonal than personal, some active, most passive.	Encourage informal time to get to know one another.
Uncertain about team membership.	New team—discuss and agree on core and secondary team membership. New team member—mentor should discuss and ensure understanding.
Conflict is neither discussed nor addressed.	Encourage conflict recognition as an opportunity for creative problem solving.

Phase II: Norming

Symptoms	Interventions
Difficult to understand goals and purpose of the team.	Discuss the goals as a team.
Attempt to establish common team goals.	Discuss and agree as a team.
Mistrust each other; exhibit caution and conformity.	Structure opportunities for informal communication about training, values, experience, and duties of each member.
Begin to see role overlaps.	Observe members from other disciplines; discuss overlaps.
Know conflicts are present; cover them up or whitewash them.	Encourage conflict recognition as an opportunity for creative problem solving.
A few members attempt to establish bonds with others who have similar views.	Form a subcommittee and include members from different coalitions.
Team establishes ground rules; begins to clarify common roles.	Reinforce ground rules; negotiate common roles.
Team may want leader(s) to assume responsibility.	Identify informal leadership roles that need to be filled and who can fill them.
Team tries strategies to increase equality of leadership (e.g., rotating leaders).	Emphasize development of competence for different leadership roles.

(*Continued*)

Table 5.2   (*Continued*)

Phase II: Norming

Symptoms	Interventions
Defensive communication and disruptive behavior increases.	At process team meeting, give open feedback and discuss patterns of disruption and solutions.
Team members are frustrated.	Promote informal leadership for resolving problems.
Some members project blame and responsibility toward the perceived leaders.	Promote informal leadership for resolving problems.
Team members compete.	Discuss different leadership roles; praise members for individual contributions.
Some members come to meetings late or do not attend them.	Review rules for membership (e.g., attendance at meetings, start and end meetings on time, ignore late arrivals).

Phase III: Confronting

Symptoms	Interventions
Can no longer avoid conflicts; some members verbally attack other members.	Bring team conflicts to team forum or process leader (if identified); process leader mediates between individuals.
Conflicts of leadership, equality, commitment increase.	Identify, clarify, and assign informal leadership roles.
Members feel anxiety over expression of affect.	Encourage expressions of affect—positive and negative.
Address some conflicts directly.	Encourage the practice of constructive confrontation; focus on solutions to problems.
Some members withdraw from the team.	Review reasons for leaving; may be a symptom of team dysfunction.
Search for leader who will resolve conflicts.	Identify members with skills and willingness to assume role of process analyzer.
Functional leaders emerge.	Identify and encourage informal leaders.
Realize that power is not equal.	Identify all potential power sources.
Realize that everyone has power for leadership and decision making.	Encourage members to recognize and assume power sources they are capable of assuming.
Conflicts lead to constructive confrontation.	Help the team (members) discuss and resolve conflicts; regard as opportunity for creative problem solving.
Team reclarifies goals and roles.	As a team, update goals; discuss roles and agree.
Form coalitions that change according to needs of the team.	Praise this as a sign of the team's growth.

Phase IV: Performing

Symptoms	Interventions
Appreciate differences of members.	Encourage this behavior.
Members encourage and help each other.	Reinforce helping behaviors as part of team's culture.
Increase reality testing; team grows stronger.	Schedule open feedback of members to team.
The norm is self-initiated active participation.	Praise informal leadership.
Members trust each other and develop strong relationships.	Enjoy; offer to mentor new members.
Members meet regularly and come on time.	Reinforce as part of team culture.
See conflicts as normal and use as impetus for program improvement.	Reinforce as part of team culture.
Emphasize productivity and problem solving.	Reinforce as part of team culture.
Members responsible for leadership in teaching, wherever skills warrant it.	Reinforce as part of team culture; ensure all informal leadership roles are filled.

Phase V: Leaving

Individual leaves

Symptoms	Interventions
Individual may feel anger or sadness toward members or the team in general.	Praise the member for team accomplishments; wish members well in new endeavor.
Members deny impending departure because of disbelief and regret.	As a team, discuss interim situation; plan for replacement.
Team expresses wish for member to remain with the team.	Accept as a sign of a significant loss to team; regard as potential ghost for team to address in the future.
Team may regress to an earlier phase.	Determine the team's developmental phase; proceed from there.
Individual may express happiness over leaving the team.	Accept that the member is happy and that the team has a shortage to address.

Team terminates

Symptoms	Interventions
Some members withdraw; depression and sadness result.	Develop a team plan of action; develop a personal plan of action.
Members express team's superiority.	Celebrate and record the team's accomplishments.
Express feelings as testimonials.	Listen and encourage team members to express their feelings and plan for their future.
Affirm team membership as valuable.	Celebrate with an eye to the future.

phase. Team members who are new to an existing IHT go through the *forming* phase at various rates. The rates depend on the amount and quality of their prior team experience, how quickly they engage with a group, how actively they want to learn the ways of the team, and how quickly the other team members expect them to assume a given role. If the IHT has already developed an early culture of "getting to work and ignoring conflict," the newer team members will likely act in the same manner.

Norming Phase

In groups, the second phase of development is the conflict or storming phase. Healthcare professionals generally do not wish to or are not given the time to work through their conflicts. They are expected to get to work. Thus, in this model the first recurring phase is *norming*. This direct move into *norming* interferes with questioning and might place the team in a *groupthink* mentality. Conflict arises, and while task conflicts might be addressed, more significant team conflicts, like having a team member who does not have the skills to do the job, are pushed under the table in the *norming* phase. This causes frustration to build as this phase progresses, and, rather than addressing the team problems, members have a tendency to retreat into their comfortable discipline-specific ways of operating. It is common for healthcare teams to become stuck in this phase. Many IHTs never progress beyond *norming,* because healthcare practitioners do not like conflict and use many excuses for avoiding it. If the team encounters a lot of change and does not address significant team conflicts, it is continually recycled back into the early *norming* phase.

As the *norming* phase progresses, it is common for IHTs to strive for equality of leadership. Teams may initiate rotating leadership for various tasks, irrespective of the qualifications and constraints of individual members. The team might ignore the fact that the pharmacist does not have the skills or desire to run the team meeting, or that the physician does not have the time to do the preparatory work. The team expects them to take turns with the rest of the team's members. Competition between disciplines might also occur, based on expectations of equality. Since there is role overlap between health professions, members from different disciplines might vie to interview a particular patient, insist on being the first to see a patient in clinic, or question whether it is the social worker's role to call a nursing director or whether it is the nurse's role to check on a placement for a client. The conflict becomes more difficult to keep under the table as the team approaches the *confronting* phase.

Confronting Phase

Conflict erupts and is addressed in the *confronting* phase. Whether the team confronts the conflict in a constructive manner or not will dictate whether the team moves on to the *performing* phase. The early part of the *confronting* phase can be quite uncomfortable for the team. The emergence of conflict might frighten some members, who move back to the overtly more comfortable *norming* phase where conflict is usually covered up. In the *confronting* phase, members realize the power of constructive confrontation and use the opportunity to engage in problem-solving behavior. As informal leaders emerge, there is a realization that, although every member must have power for decision making, the power is not equal. As members realize their potential for power, it enables the assumption of informal leadership roles by each member of the team.

The IHT begins to move into the *performing* phase when individual members demonstrate their power in the process of collaboration. Members might also protect the rights of their fellow members to use power. By establishing the right to individual power as a norm, the team ensures that a few members do not assume all of the power, and that every member has power for decision making. When this occurs, constructive confrontation becomes a team norm. The initial team goals and roles should be reexamined (perhaps with heated debate) in this phase. Reexamining goals and roles may involve an increase in disruptive behavior. The team's approach to the inevitable conflict depends on its maturity level and the conflict and decision making styles of the team's members. Each time this occurs, the team builds on prior history and reestablishes itself with more depth and maturity.

Performing Phase

The team is *performing* when the conflicts are directed more at program development than at individual members. Every conflict becomes an opportunity to learn and improve the way the team does its work. Also, the differences of each team member become an appreciated addition to the team. Members trust each other enough to view conflicts as normal and essential to further team development. This tends to be a phase that teams visit occasionally. When there are constant and intense changes in a healthcare system, IHTs usually do not remain in this phase for long periods.

Leaving Phase

The *leaving* phase may not be included in some team models. Although this phase is intermittent, it is an important part of a team's development because it is normal for IHTs to have some turnover. Leaving might be temporary or permanent and might involve one or many members; some of those members will be powerful team leaders, and some will be members with limited capacity for team function. The qualities of the leaving members will be reflected in how much the team grieves or denies the changes that take place as the member exits. Occasionally, the entire team can be threatened with termination as an organization chooses to downsize. In such cases, there can be a powerful effect on the entire organization as the team's members choose different methods to cope with their loss.

Individual and Team Movement through the Phases

Both the ongoing team members and the entire team might continue to recycle through any of the phases of team development as they encounter personal or professional problems or as the team encounters change. It is important to note that individual team members and the team itself might all be in different phases of development. Also, team members are not always accurate in judging their individual and the team's phases of development. Longer-term team members tend to be less accurate in judging their phase of development in relation to the team.[7]

Tables 5.1 and 5.2 are complementary to Figures 5.1 through 5.4. The stick people in the figures represent team members as they proceed through the phases of team development. The figures depict numerous features of this team development model, for example, team vs. individual development, differing developmental phases, direction of movement, rate of movement, newer vs. longer-term team members, and flatness (Figures 5.1 and 5.2) vs. depth (Figures 5.3 and 5.4) of team culture.

Because individual team members do not always join a team at the same time, some members find themselves in a phase of development different from the rest of the team. Another reason for this differential development of individual and team is the varying amount of time that some members are assigned to the team. Full-time team members might engage more rapidly with the team. Some individuals are more likely than others to enjoy working on a team. Other individuals might just take a long time to trust others. And, individuals who were sent to the team against their

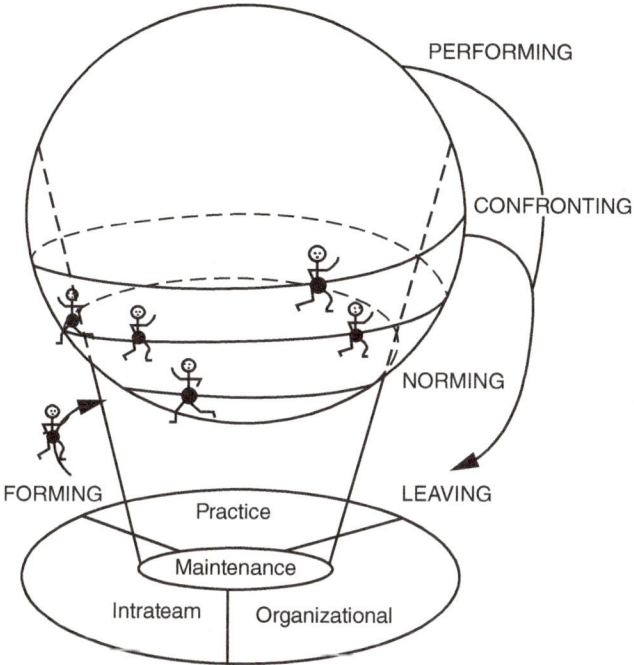

Figure 5.1　**Emerging Interprofessional Healthcare Team in the Norming Phase**

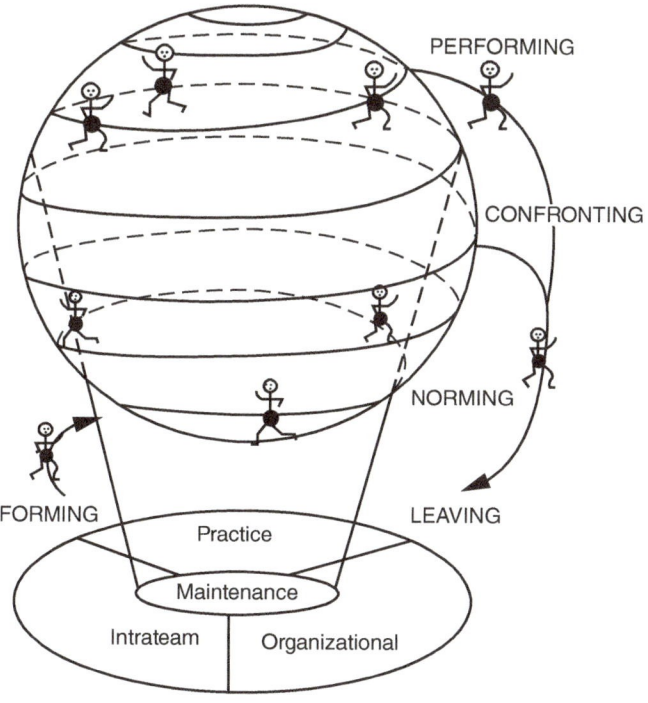

Figure 5.2　**Ongoing Poorly Developed Healthcare Team Struggling to Survive**

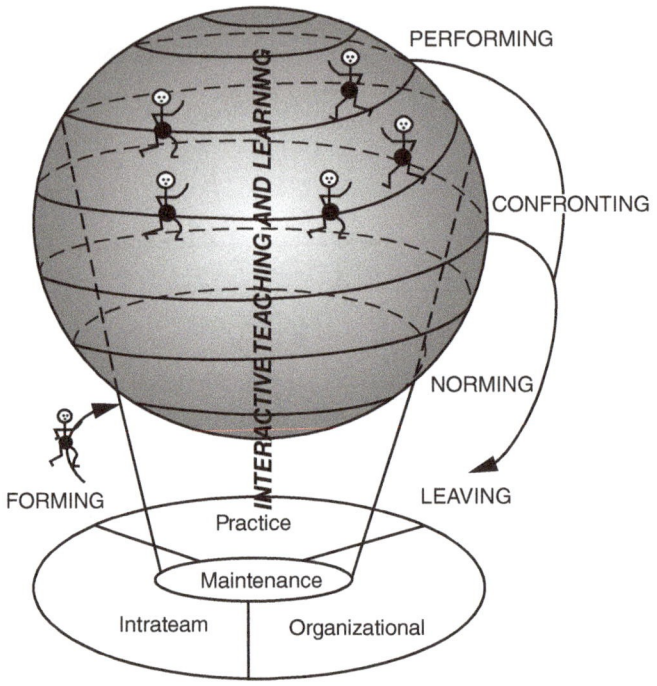

Figure 5.3 **Well-Functioning Interprofessional Healthcare Team**

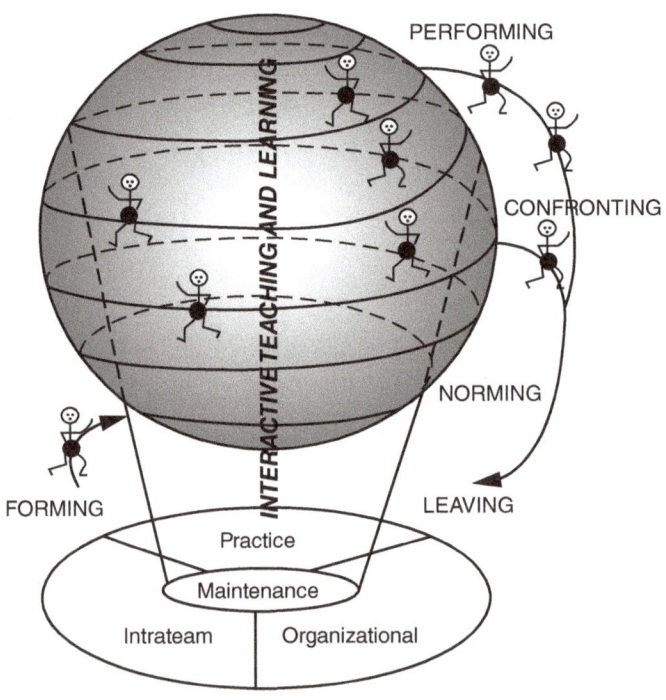

Figure 5.4 **Interprofessional Healthcare Team in Chaos**

desires may never progress beyond the *forming* or the *norming* phases. It is important for team members to watch for other members who are having difficulty assimilating into the team, so they can offer support and possible assistance. Teams, especially long-term ones, may have some members in each phase of team development, as in Figure 5.4. This makes it difficult to determine the true phase of the team. A mature team in this situation is probably in chaos, and members should use this chaos as an indication that they need to engage in some formal team restructuring.

Team members can proceed in different directions and at different rates through the model, dependent on changing practice and intrateam and organizational factors. The team components and phases of development as depicted in Tables 5.1 and 5.2 are the influences that spark successes or failures in the team. Each member of the team can recognize or ignore the ever-changing team components in Table 5.1. Each member can view these team components as either positive or negative stresses. The prevalent perceptions draw individual members and the entire team either up toward *performing* as in Figure 5.3 or down toward *norming* as in Figure 5.1.

Each stick person represents the phase of a member. The phase that contains the majority of stick figures is the current phase of the team (e.g., the team in Figure 5.1 is in the *norming* phase). The larger stick figures represent team members who have been with the team for more than a year, and the smaller stick figures represent members who have been with the team for less than a year. A larger stick person in the *forming* or *norming* phase as in Figure 5.1 would indicate a longer-term team member who may be working within their discipline but who is not engaged with the team. A smaller stick person in the *confronting* or *performing* phase, as in Figure 5.4, would indicate a member who recently joined the team, quickly engaged with the team, and rapidly moved through the phases. A team member who rapidly advances through the phases is likely someone who was trained to work on an IHT, has worked on IHTs in the past, or has leadership characteristics that are important to the team.

This model is dynamic in that it reflects the growing depth and resilience of an established team. A newly forming IHT, without a sense of history, would be depicted as a unidimensional flat entity as in Figure 5.1. In this team, all of the stick people are in either the *forming* or the *norming* phases. They have not yet begun to constructively confront difficult team conflicts. Figure 5.2 represents an ongoing IHT that has some longer-term members. Some members who are performing in relation to the team are likely informal leaders. However, the team has not begun to address its conflicts, and although some members are in the performing phase, the team has no cultural depth. One longer-term member is leaving (perhaps out of frustration), and newer members appear somewhat confused about their position in relation to the team.

An IHT that has proceeded through the first three or four phases at least once takes on a multidimensional quality. It establishes a history and culture that helps it to reexamine new questions with a background of experience. If all members feel empowered to assume appropriate leadership, the team has the capacity to learn and grow, using past mistakes to feed new ideas. The team represented in Figure 5.3 has a depth of culture that has come from working through its problems in an open and constructive manner. It is a healthy team moving toward performing. In contrast, the team in Figure 5.4 has probably experienced major recent changes. As stated earlier, it is a team in chaos. However, because it has a depth of culture, it should be able to quickly recognize its problems and develop strategies for addressing them. Depending on the extent of the changes and the loss of its leaders, a mature team might temporarily move to the *norming* phase before it recovers.

IHTs may not always follow a specific order of development, *or* development may occur so quickly that the sequence is imperceptible. After *forming*, IHTs may quickly establish norms, because they are under pressure to perform. However, these initial norms often promote discipline-specific goals and do not ensure good outcomes for complex problems. Some IHTs might remain in a static state of *norming* for long periods of time. On the other hand, an IHT might proceed directly from *norming* to *performing*, especially when its members are experienced at working with other disciplines. It is probable that such a team has not been challenged by conflict, and even though well-functioning, it does not possess the depth of culture to survive over time. Additionally, it is common for newer teams to view themselves as *performing* when it is clear that they avoid the constructive use of conflict and have little depth of culture. The current phase of the IHT may not denote the depth of the team's development, because a well-developed team may temporarily revert to the *norming* phase. If the team has leaders who are in more advanced phases, it should quickly recover and increase its depth.

It is interesting to speculate about the team in this case, what phase of development the team and its members might be in, and whether this team has any depth to its development. Some of the other issues to consider are whether this team has an interprofessional definition of the patient's problems, what are the appropriate roles and tasks for nursing and social work, how team members might build more trust, and what other team-related problems might be relevant to this situation.

BOX 5.1   A CASE OF MISCOMMUNICATION OR OF POOR TEAM FUNCTION?

A social worker on a clinical outreach team with several nurses discovered that a patient of hers had fallen the previous day. The nurse, the only team member to be alerted, had found someone to stay with the patient but had not informed the social worker of this. This effort had taken the nurse many hours, and, because she also had nursing visits to make, she ended up working until 9 p.m. In speaking with the patient about placement in a group home, the nurse discovered that the patient wanted placement in a new group home that was near her home. The nurse promised the patient that she would try to place her in that home and called to begin the arrangements. She found that the outreach program did not have a contract with the new home for payment and also had no information on the quality of the home.

The social worker for the clinical outreach team was not contacted until late the next morning when the nurse asked about using the new group home. The social worker told the nurse of the difficulty, and the nurse continued to stress how important it was for this client to be close to her home and that the client was really counting on it. The social worker told the nurse to ask their supervisor to make an exception and offered alternatives if the new group home did not work out. The supervisor refused the request, and they placed the patient in an alternative home, which felt all right to the social worker because she anticipated that the client would return home after two weeks. If the stay were to be permanent, the social worker would have tried harder; but because it was a crisis, she sensed that they should take what was available. The social worker felt that if she had been involved on the first day, the place close to the patient's home would never have been offered, because she knew the agency had temporarily stopped establishing new group home providers. She could have helped prevent the nurse from working late by assisting with the planning.

Additionally, when the social worker talked to the daughter the day after the fall, the daughter said she felt bad that no one called her or her brother on the day of the fall. She was upset and her confidence in the program had been shaken. The daughter had requested to be called if something really serious happened to her mother. The social worker apologized that no one had called and assured her they would call in the future. The social worker knew that had she been informed earlier, she would have notified the daughter, because it is easier for two people to think of all the important details. Also, the social worker considered contacting family members as an important part of her job.

Achieving Efficiency: Matrix of Interprofessional Problem Solving

Efficiency involves time, resources, cost, and long-term outcomes. Healthcare organizations have traditionally measured short-term and focused outcomes (e.g., length of visits, numbers of patients seen by each discipline, or correctly dispensing a prescription). Longer-term global health outcomes (which may represent a greater initial cost)—maintaining independent function, patient follow-through on treatment regimens, iatrogenic effects, and effects on family and caregivers—have often been ignored. Healthcare organizations continue to measure short-term focused outcomes because these organizations are based on a business production paradigm and are reimbursed for this type of outcome. Unfortunately, looking at short-term and focused outcomes usually does not work with complex and ambiguous problems.

If healthcare organizations have difficulty measuring long-term global outcomes, it is no wonder they have difficulty measuring the efficiency of teamwork. Hiring team members and providing initial team training is not sufficient to ensure that a team will perform. In fact, if the components of a team are in place and the team is well on its way toward the *performing* phase, it still might not be efficient in its problem solving. If team members do not know whether or not to involve other team members, which members to involve in discussions, and when to involve them, the team might unknowingly be using more resources than it needs to use. To become efficient, the team must direct the interplay between individual disciplines and the organization of the team as these relate to the types of problems team members encounter. Team members must learn to define the scope of a problem in a way that is neither too narrow nor too broad, identify the fewest disciplines needed to address the problem well, and prioritize the assessments and interventions that are necessary to address the problem. Tables 5.3 and 5.4 might be useful

Table 5.3   **Efficiency Estimates for Effects of Six Variables on Interprofessional Intervention When a Problem Is Tame**

	Appropriate Disciplines	Inappropriate Disciplines	
Greater Than One Discipline	Low	Low	Highly Organized
One Discipline	High	Low	Low Organization

Table 5.4   **Efficiency Estimates for Effects of Six Variables on Interprofessional Intervention When a Problem Is Wicked**

	Appropriate Disciplines	Inappropriate Disciplines	
Greater Than One Discipline	High	Low	Highly Organized
One Discipline	Low	Low	Low Organization

for suggesting ways to increase the efficiency of interprofessional problem solving.

Tame versus Wicked Problems

Tame problems are those that can be defined. The outcome can be predicted and procedures for intervention can be quantified, measured, and replicated. Administering an influenza vaccination, diagnosing a simple cold or the stomach flu in a 10-year-old, treating an infected cut in a healthy person, and following up an uncomplicated gall bladder surgery are all relatively tame problems. They can and should be efficiently accomplished by one provider or a small set of providers (see Table 5.3).

Increasingly, healthcare systems have attempted to create standardized methods and procedures for addressing tame and recurring problems. Many of those systems and procedures have evolved from efficiency models created by corporations. However, it is more difficult to standardize efficiency and effectiveness approaches for complex situations that are also uncommon. Those situations require highly trained professionals who are nimble at assessing and targeting expertise that is appropriate to a particular situation.

Wicked problems are the opposite of tame. The term "wicked problem" was used by Rittel and Webber[8] and aptly captures the complexity and ambiguity that are inherent in many patient and team problems. In health care, a wicked problem is one that is difficult to formulate, has more than one explanation, is often a symptom of another problem, is frequently unique, and does not resolve with a simple intervention. Such a problem is multifaceted, and many of those facets are intentionally or unintentionally hidden. The following are some examples of potentially wicked problems: scheduling an influenza vaccination in a demented elder who has had a prior adverse reaction to an influenza vaccine, treating a cryptosporidium infection presenting as stomach flu and rheumatoid arthritis in a person recovering from cancer treatments, treating an infected cut in a diabetic patient with poor vision who lives alone in a house with no running water, or evaluating a patient whose spouse reports a sudden radical change in behavior. In order to achieve high efficiency, each of these cases will require input from more than one discipline (see Table 5.4).

There is a continuum that exists between wicked and tame problems, and it is critical for practitioners to learn to accurately assess where a problem lies on the continuum. In the middle of the continuum lie moderate problems that may also call for more than one discipline. When the patient repeatedly returns with the same problem or when the patient is frail or in jeopardy, the problem moves further over to the wicked end of the scale. Assessing the type of problem is one of the most difficult aspects of interprofessional problem solving. It requires a realization by practitioners that one cannot solve the problem alone. It also requires open dialogue with members of more than one discipline. A clinician who is taught autonomous practice will look at the presenting problem through her own discipline-specific glasses and ignore potentially helpful perspectives from others. Consequently, the clinician can miss the significance of a wicked problem and might ignore the potential for other disciplines to help solve the problem. In the interest of team efficiency, practitioners must be taught how to recognize and treat both tame and wicked problems.

Box 5.2   Words of Advice

Observing how an IHT assesses and treats a wicked problem is a good indicator of the depth of the team's interprofessional culture and of the efficiency and effectiveness of the team.

Using Appropriate Disciplines

Whether the problem is tame or wicked, having the appropriate team members address it is a key to attaining efficiency on an IHT. If the problem is tame and one person can handle it, that person should be the team member who is most expert in that particular area. This requires that team members know their own competencies and have an awareness of the core knowledge base of other disciplines. It also entails knowing how different disciplines frame problems and problem solve. For example, faced with a brittle case of juvenile diabetes, a physician might frame the problem as a need to titrate medication and monitor glucose levels. A nurse might frame the problem as a need for family education and ongoing monitoring. A social worker might frame the problem as one of educating peers and caregiver stress. There are obvious overlaps in the three ways of framing this problem, because "monitoring" might involve patient, caregiver, and perhaps peers. Since this case of juvenile diabetes presents as a wicked problem, it might take all three disciplines working together to frame the problem so that they can more efficiently resolve it.

How different disciplines are taught or not taught to work with practitioners from other disciplines is a major factor in whether they use the talents of other disciplines to help solve wicked problems. If practitioners from a certain discipline are taught to demonstrate an authoritarian leadership style, it will be difficult for them to engage the willing services of other disciplines. If practitioners from another discipline are always expected to defer to other more highly trained practitioners, it will hinder their willingness to offer constructive ideas for care. If practitioners from a given discipline are taught to "do their own thing" without taking into account the input of other practitioners, that is what they will do. All of this affects the economics of team practice.

Every discipline has areas of overlap with other disciplines. Practitioners frequently take advantage of areas of overlap by assuming duties that might be considered more in the domain of another profession. For example, a general medical nurse or an occupational therapist might attempt some assessment and intervention of a patient's depression. For mild cases this will work fine. However, if the patient's depression is complicated by a long-standing personality disorder, occasional manic episodes, or a failing marriage, the clinician may be in over his or her head without realizing it. The clinicians in this case should know the core competencies of psychiatry, psychology, and social work, and should call in the appropriate discipline(s). The patient's problems might best respond to a plan by the occupational therapist, social worker, and psychiatrist. In this case, the nurse would bow out for the time being.

A busy nurse who has some skill in identifying resources to support a patient in the community may be out of his or her league when those resources depend on uncertain funding sources, an area in which the social worker is current. A social worker who realizes a family is living on junk food might speak with family members about their eating habits, but if the problem is serious a dietitian could counsel the family more efficiently and with greater impact. These examples point out the value of understanding the skills of other disciplines that enable the practitioner to call in a more appropriate practitioner before a situation consumes limited resources.

It is also important for practitioners to learn the difference between professional competencies and other learned competencies that team members might have. A nursing assistant might be good at listening to a patient's problems and at giving that patient sound advice. When that nursing assistant leaves and is replaced by another, it would be common for members of other disciplines to expect the replacement to have the same counseling skills as the previous nursing assistant, when, in fact, it is not one of the job skills for that position. There is also a difference between competencies and personalities. For example, team members might expect that all social workers will project a sense of protecting the self-determination of the client or that all nurses will exhibit very caring behavior toward clients. While some of these behaviors are built into each profession, there is wide latitude in behaviors that are exercised by virtue of different personalities.

Knowing the core competencies of different disciplines and the levels within each discipline is critical not only for members of IHTs, but also for healthcare administrators. In order to hire and/or engage the correct disciplines, an administrator must know what each discipline is expected to do well. An administrator will need this knowledge to communicate with internal and external funding sources about the needs of the clients and the best way to meet those needs.

There are also gray areas of discipline knowledge, areas that individuals trained in a particular discipline know something about but are not expert in. Physicians as a profession used to dwell heavily in those gray areas. In recent years, that role has been increasingly assumed by PAs, NPs, and RNs. With cost containment and limited funding for dealing with wicked problems, the discipline that takes responsibility for coordination and integration of care needs to question whether dwelling in all of the gray areas of health care delivers the most efficient and effective patient care. Administrators have readily accepted nursing in these roles, because it leads them to believe they can eliminate other disciplines and reap cost savings by doing so. However, no one discipline can do everything well and efficiently, especially when dealing with wicked problems. Accepting a discipline as a universal provider confuses other disciplines. It can also confuse the discipline that is accepting that role, because that discipline is more likely to define a wicked problem as tame. This is a natural reflex, since tame problems are easier to address. The intent here is to raise this issue as something that has the potential to affect any discipline and that can interfere with the effectiveness and efficiency of patient care and interprofessional practice.

Calling in another discipline when there is a wicked problem in a gray area requires more than consulting with that discipline. If the problem is a wicked one, it will require a dialogue and joint action between individuals from several disciplines. To achieve maximum efficiency, there will need to be a system of identifying such problems so that a variety of disciplines can relate to them. Additionally, the team needs a mechanism for identifying the presenting problem and allied problems in relation to an integrated goal (i.e., frame it as an interprofessional problem). The team can then create stepped-in procedures for different disciplines to move in and out of the maze as it moves the patient toward long-term resolution.

Level of Team Organization Required

The efficiency of an IHT hinges on defragmenting the structure and processes involved in the assessment and care plan. One of the early tasks of an IHT should be to structure and/or agree on a unified assessment and treatment process. As part of this process, the team needs to establish the procedures for charting progress notes related to the interprofessional treatment plan. This exercise will have a profound impact on the development of a new IHT. It forces members to discuss their discipline-specific roles, what their roles might be in relation to the team, areas of overlap between the different disciplines, and how to frame wicked problems as interprofessional problems. Continuing its development, a team should move on to discussing and adapting its standards of practice and critical pathways for common and recurring patient problems. If this is done in the context of the team's unified assessment and treatment structure and process, the team will be well on its way to performing and delivering excellent care.

There are many different types of team meetings. Patient care meetings can be for the purpose of organizing, framing problems, discussing problems, or reviewing and revising approaches to problems. Teams also need team-building meetings, regular meetings to review their progress as a team, and meetings to address problems that impede the function of the team. Teams often ignore meetings related to their function, either because team members are afraid of conflict or because administrators do not value these meetings and do not allow time for them.

Organizing the team's structure and process for different types of meetings is part of the efficiency of teams. Staff will either model or avoid the types of meetings they have been exposed to in the past. Just because the team decides to stand up during meetings or restrict the time for presenters does not ensure those meetings will be useful or efficient. If an agenda item is not a wicked problem, it probably does not belong on the agenda. If meetings are ill planned, begin late, and have little focus, busy providers will learn to avoid them at all costs. On the other hand, if team members experience well-run interprofessional meetings that start and end on time, involve the right mix of disciplines, are run by a qualified meeting leader, are focused, and encourage dialogue about difficult issues, they will model those types of meetings within and across team boundaries.

An IHT needs protocols and procedures for members to act, react, and interact with each other on a continuous basis, not just at weekly staff meetings. Achieving similar mental models of the team's mission and the tasks that team members need to perform should allow the team to function more effectively.[9] Framing and expressing problems, not as discreet entities but as pieces of an integrated whole, are essential aspects of the efficient IHT. As team members learn about the scope of knowledge and problem-solving abilities of other disciplines, they can efficiently utilize the overlaps between one another.[10] However, these achievements are only the basic foundation for a mature IHT. When team members can use their team knowledge to capitalize on each other's reflexive or intuitive problem-solving behaviors, they will advance to creatively and efficiently solve wicked problems.[11] As the team's mental models become more highly developed, they might even help the team sustain itself during times of chaotic organizational change.[12]

Just because numerous disciplines are relevant to a wicked problem does not mean that they all have to physically evaluate the patient. In an IHT that is highly organized, one or two disciplines might be responsible for conducting an initial assessment. Some of the disciplines would advise a smaller core team on how to handle the problem. Questioning

---

Box 5.3   Words of Advice

Interprofessional healthcare teams must be highly organized entities. If an IHT is not organized and functional, there is no possibility that its full talents can be used when needed.

Box 5.4   Paradox of Interprofessional Thinking

Interprofessional thinking involves the maximum amount of autonomy with the least amount of anarchy (turmoil). Turmoil can come
from the patient, the family, the system, coworkers, other disciplines, and the team, and it can come from within oneself.

---

and teaching would flow freely across disciplines. In the case of a family
living on junk food, the dietitian might just advise the social worker until
the social worker established enough trust so that the family would agree
to interact directly with the dietitian.

Every practitioner encounters situations on a daily basis that require
intervention by one discipline. Practitioners also encounter situations that
require a highly organized team. If the resources of an entire team are used
to engage tame problems, it is not an efficient use of resources and is seen
by practitioners as a waste of time (see Table 5.3). On the other hand, if no
team is available to address wicked problems, it is not only inefficient (see
Table 5.4), but also can be very costly and frustrating for the practitioner
and the client. Learning to distinguish the type of structure needed for a
given situation is a skill that must be acquired by practitioners. Learning
how much and what kinds of structures are needed to address different
types of problems are critical skills for an IHT.

Methods of Team Practice

Some practitioners erroneously believe that being a member of an IHT
means they must give up autonomous practice or, conversely, that most
decisions should be brought to the team. Although most health care practice is autonomous, health professionals must also be able to recognize

when a complex situation calls for input from members of their own or other disciplines. In fact, autonomous practice is one of at least six methods of team practice:

1. Autonomous;
2. The *ad hoc group* or *task group,* which meets to work on a specific issue and then disbands;
3. The *formal work group* that is ongoing and consists of professionals from one discipline;
4. The *formal work group* of many disciplines;
5. The *one-discipline interactive team* that works on its developmental processes; and
6. The *interactive team* that is interprofessional.

A family practitioner working regularly with a gastroenterologist and a psychiatrist serving patients with eating disorders would be using a unidisciplinary method of practice, because they are all physicians and have formalized their process. If they provide information to one another and each make independent decisions, they would be using a formal unidisciplinary work group method. If they are interdependent, have defined team protocols, openly discuss options, and reflect on their teamwork, they are an interactive unidisciplinary team. If the family practitioner also worked regularly with a clinical nurse specialist, social worker, and dietitian, they would be using either multidisciplinary or interprofessional methods of team practice. If they provide information to one another and each make independent decisions, they would be using a formal multidisciplinary work group method. If they are interdependent, openly discuss options, and reflect on their teamwork, they are an interactive interprofessional team. If any or all of these professionals talked briefly together occasionally and/or informally, they would be using an ad hoc task group method of teamwork. Each method of team practice has specific characteristics that are specified in Table 5.5.

There are advantages and disadvantages to each of the methods of team practice. The *ad hoc group* might be the appropriate method to rapidly address a unique problem with implications for the larger organization. However, because solutions of the *ad hoc group* often lack breadth and depth, it might not be an effective method for addressing complex ongoing practice issues. The multidisciplinary formal work group might be a good method for discussing routine health care that

Table 5.5 Methods of Interprofessional Healthcare Practice

	Description	Advantages	Disadvantages
Ad Hoc/Task Group	• ≥ One discipline/department/agency • Group selects or agrees on a leader • Rules set by the group • Solves a problem and disbands	• Focus on one issue • No elaborate rules • Quick and may be effective for well defined problem • Members capture enthusiasm	• Solutions often lack depth/breadth • Some fear expressing views • Low status may hinder openness • Difficulty getting together
Formal Unidisciplinary Work Group (e.g., MDs from multiple specialties)	• One discipline/department/ ≥ One agency • Members report to group • Individual identities more important than integrated diagnoses • Don't work on team problems • Leadership by election or rank • Discipline-specific care	• Members speak same language • Final decisions by formal leader • Ongoing • Rules established to keep order • Security of one discipline • Solutions often have depth	• Some resent leaders decisions • Solutions lack breadth • May miss important problems • Little integrative dialogue • Inefficient with complexity
Formal Multidisciplinary Work Group (e.g., MD, RN, SW, OT)	• ≥ One discipline/department/ ≥ One agency • Members report to group • Individual identities more important than integrated diagnoses • Don't work on team problems • Leadership by election or rank • Discipline-specific care	• Final decisions by formal leader • Ongoing • Rules established to keep order • Information from many perspectives • Solutions may have breadth	• Some resent leaders decisions • Speak different languages • Solutions not integrated • Full court press by each discipline overwhelms patient • Little integrative dialogue • Inefficient with complexity

(Continued)

Table 5.5 *(Continued)*

	Description	Advantages	Disadvantages
Interactive Unidisciplinary Team (e.g., MDs from multiple specialties)	• One discipline/department/ ≥ One agency • Integrated diagnoses • Team goals for patient and team • Members interdependent • Team structures enable collaboration • Work on team problems • Leadership appropriate to issue/expertise	• Members speak same language • Share responsibility for leadership • More openness • More informal collaboration • Solutions have depth • Members feel empowered • Culture encourages creativity	• Initial decisions take more time • Solutions lack breadth • May miss important problems • Need time and space to discuss values; renegotiate roles, leadership, conflict
Interactive Interprofessional Team (e.g., MD, RN, SW, OT)	• ≥ One discipline/department/ ≥ One agency • Integrated diagnoses • Team goals for patient and team • Members interdependent • Team structures enable collaboration • Work on team problems • Leadership appropriate to issue/expertise	• Integrated efficient care • Share responsibility for leadership • Solutions address complex problems • Solutions have depth and breadth • Members feel empowered • Creative approaches to complexity • Understand autonomous practice	• Initial decisions take more time • Members must learn different languages/terms • Effort to maintain the team • Need time and space to clarify values; renegotiate roles, leadership, conflict
Autonomous Practice	• Individual decides based on knowledge	• Quick, appropriate solutions to simple and/or common problems	• Works only if clinician understands interprofessional practice

needs to involve input from many disciplines. However, because solutions from this method often lack depth, it is not an effective method for addressing complex issues that have no single solution and that tend to be ongoing.

When healthcare practitioners encounter a problem, whether patient-related or not, they have a decision to make. They can solve the problem alone or use one of the other forms of team practice. The choice of whether to contact someone else, who to contact and when, depends on their philosophy of practice, level of training, and security in opening themselves to another point of view. If a given situation calls for the skills of a single profession and a person from that profession feels comfortable applying those skills, he or she will likely work independently.

If a situation is seen as demanding skills a professional doesn't have, he or she might consult another professional, either from the same or another discipline. The discipline that is chosen will depend on availability, potential of saving time, and the individual's knowledge of what that discipline has to offer. It will also involve some degree of trust, meaning that a professional needs to know something about the person he or she is contacting, such as knowledge base, values, methods of gathering and processing information, perceived accuracy, reliability, and speed of delivery. The practitioner might also assume, based on past experience or training, that a particular profession or department should be able to handle certain problems. This knowledge and past experience with another provider is the basis of trust and provides practitioners with the sense that their requests will be heeded.

If we do not know the capabilities of other healthcare professionals, our expectations for them will be inaccurate. Credentials are not always sufficient as predictors of a practitioner's knowledge. While it is essential to have an awareness of the expected knowledge base of the different levels within a profession, it is also very helpful to know how someone was trained. If we think we know what a healthcare professional should know (based only on their credentials), and ask someone of that profession for help on a case, then we may be dissatisfied with the results, and will likely exclude that person from further dialogue.

For example, we may think that a registered nurse should be able to suggest interventions for a patient who has a borderline personality disorder, cardiac insufficiency, chronic pain from rheumatoid arthritis, caregiver burden from caring for her demented spouse, and is not complying with her medications. If the registered nurse is a clinician with a master's degree, we would probably be correct in assuming that he or she could understand the issues. If the registered nurse has a two-year nursing degree and little experience, we will likely be disappointed with the interaction and consequently may decide to tackle the problem ourselves, even though it could be done more efficiently with the help of a well-trained nurse.

Alternately, we may choose to speak with a member of our own discipline because we have more trust in what to expect, even though this may be an inefficient use of our time. We may also waste time trying to contact a busy physician when we could have more efficiently asked an appropriately trained and lesser-paid nurse. We might also have asked a clinical pharmacist. These are typical decisions in everyday practice for all healthcare practitioners. And yet, we are seldom taught to make these choices. Instead we are taught to function in the "safe" world of our own narrow practice range.

While health professionals recognize the need to interact with others in the healthcare community, it is difficult for them to do so unless they have received training in all six methods of teamwork. Healthcare practitioners cannot choose the most appropriate type of practice if they are not familiar and comfortable with their options. The six methods of team practice need to be mastered if a practitioner is to be efficient and effective. Knowing how to use one method of team practice does not assure knowing how to use another, for example, if I know how to work in an ad hoc task group, I do not necessarily know how to work in a multidisciplinary team. Learning to use the six methods of team practice is not necessarily progressive. Learning the autonomous practice of one's own discipline also does not have to precede learning about each of the other methods of team practice.

At every level of training, it is necessary for healthcare practitioners to learn the skills of interprofessional practice and the types of interaction necessary for different levels of patient problems. Learning to operate as a member of an IHT is the only way to ensure knowledge of all of the other methods of team practice. Although time-intensive, there is efficiency in training for interprofessional practice. Figure 5.5 illustrates this point. As individual practitioners and teams learn about the six methods of team practice and the most appropriate method for a given problem, they gain depth and breadth in their ability to problem solve. Both the team's members and the team become able to address increasingly complex issues. The efficiency of teamwork is achieved by correctly matching team method with the situation.

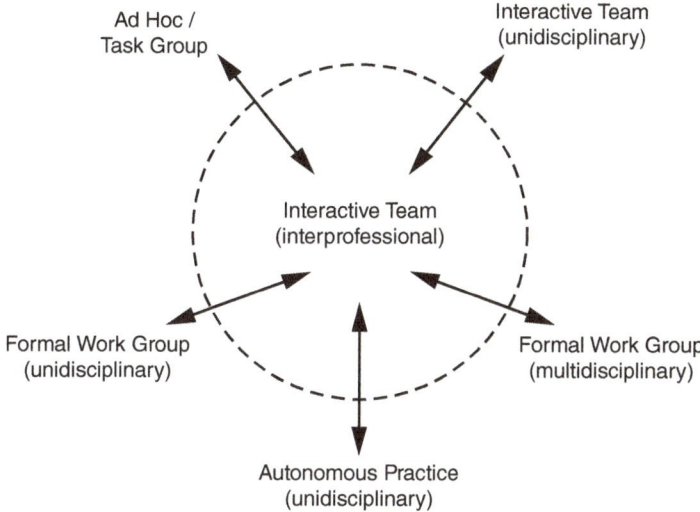

Figure 5.5   **Interprofessional Teamwork System**

Box 5.5   A Paradox of Good Health Care

To appropriately choose autonomous practice, a health practitioner must have a working knowledge of what other disciplines do and knowledge of how an interactive team operates.

Matching Problem and Practice Method

Thinking of the IHT as a fluid system of practice helps to make it more understandable. In learning efficiency within the system of interprofessional practice, all methods of team practice should be part of the arsenal of the healthcare professional. The need for ongoing interdependence and collaboration are triggers to which method of team practice is right to address a problem, whether it is related to patient care or system operation. If an IHT is to function well and be accepted as part of its broader organizational structure, it must also have the capacity to adapt to changing and complex situations.

IHTs provide structure that enables healthcare professionals to work efficiently on different types of problems. The ideal is to create a team system that allows professionals to belong to an interprofessional team, and, at the same time, use other methods of practice with individuals, teams, or groups as needs dictate. Using the model (see Figure 5.5), a physician who belonged to an IHT in a primary care clinic setting might meet briefly with a nurse and a physical therapist (ad hoc group) to discuss a hospitalized patient's needs for mobility while hospitalized. That same physician might attend a multidisciplinary planning conference (formal work group) in a long-term care facility once a week. The physician might meet monthly with a group of clinic staff physicians (unidisciplinary formal work group) to discuss policies relative to medical care. The physician might meet regularly with the other physicians who are on the interprofessional clinic team to discuss their ongoing relationship with each other and with the other health professionals on the team (unidisciplinary interactive team). The interprofessional clinic team will meet regularly to discuss patient care plans and will periodically meet to discuss the team's function.

Unfortunately, the meetings to discuss team function are often left in the dust as patient care pressures mount. Maintaining an IHT system requires strong support from both administrators and clinicians. The costs of maintaining an IHT can be easily estimated. However, those costs are usually compared to the direct costs of not maintaining an IHT. It is necessary, but more difficult, to estimate the longer-term costs of not intervening in time to avert problems. It is also necessary to estimate the cost of a team that does not function well together. Despite the difficulties

---

BOX 5.6   THE CASE OF HENRY

A cardiologist prescribed three new medications for his new patient, Henry, a 70 year old with unstable cardiac disease and hypertension. Henry told the cardiologist about his medications for diabetes but forgot to tell him about his other medications for depression and a seizure disorder that were prescribed by his family doctor. The clinic nurse gave Henry instructions for taking the three new medications. Henry procured the medicine at one pharmacy and the pharmacist gave him instructions on the medications and potential interactions between them. Henry ordered his other medications from another pharmacy that was not linked into the computer system of the first pharmacy. Some of those medications had potentially harmful interacting effects with Henry's initial medications, but he was not instructed in those side effects.

Henry was involved with a community outreach social worker who discovered that he was not taking some of his medications because they interfered with his ability to leave his home at certain times of the day so he could visit the neighborhood restaurant to eat its famous "finger-lickin' chicken" and fudge-bottom pie. Additionally, Henry forgot to take his medicine before bed, as he felt it was too difficult for him to make another trip down the stairs to get it. The social worker called a pharmacist to discuss all of the medications and to consult on a better way to fit the medication regimen into the patient's schedule. The social worker thought that consultations by an occupational therapist and a dietitian were necessary and called the clinic nurse who decided the patient needed to be seen again in the clinic. Before the patient could be scheduled, he had an acute cardiac event and was hospitalized.

of doing so, costs for each of these situations must be factored into equations for efficiency of care. Given the issues discussed in this section, it is useful to consider how the care of Henry could have been delivered more efficiently.

The reason(s) for Henry's hospitalization are unknown. However, it is logical to assume that Henry could have benefited from receiving integrated health and social care much earlier, and he would not have been receiving his medications from multiple pharmacies. If an IHT had discussed Henry's case, the recommendations of the dietitian and occupational therapist would have been woven into his treatment plan. It is possible the social worker would remain his care coordinator but would have had easy access to the rest of the team. Henry would have been integral to establishing methods for assuring his medicine was within easy reach. This case highlights that it is essential for an IHT to help specialists and external providers understand that they are part of the extended team for patients with complex problems.

Summary

Although the IHT appears to be a simple and straightforward entity, in reality it is a complex phenomenon that requires intense efforts for development and maintenance. A well-functioning IHT encompasses multiple methods of practice and achieves efficiency by applying a particular team method where and when it is needed (i.e., the least intense method required to accomplish the task).

This chapter has described a model of IHT function and maintenance. It has also outlined six methods of practice that, when understood and used, function as a system for providing efficient health care. The purpose of presenting this model is to urge you to strive for understanding rather than perfection. There is no expectation that members of an IHT will remain in the performing phase. In fact, most of the time they will probably be elsewhere. However, it is only with an understanding of the components and phases of IHT development that members of an IHT can strive to achieve the team's ideal level of practice. When properly constructed and well functioning, the IHT is a dynamic entity with ebbs and flows of development. An IHT that attends to its development and that maintains a depth of culture is not only personally rewarding to team members, but it might also be our best hope to address the situational complexity of the current healthcare system.

Initially, this model may be difficult to understand. However, it is meant to be a learning tool that you can return to as questions arise in your team development experience. Although you may not master this model the first time you read it, use it to reflect on problems that develop in the teams with which you work. Eventually, it will help you understand the complexities of those problems, and with that understanding you will be better able to devise solutions that will help your IHT develop and strengthen its practice.

IHTs continuously address problems that are both simple and complex or tame and wicked. Healthcare providers and systems can plan for problems that are tame and common. Tackling these problems can increase efficiency and satisfaction in the patient and the system's bottom line. Other problems are wicked but somewhat common, and, if identified as such, team members can construct policies and procedures to increase their efficiency in addressing these problems. However, many wicked problems are also uncommon and providing complex solutions can be costly in terms of staff time and effort. Thus, it is important to establish an IHT that can work with the broader system to improvise and effectively use the most appropriate resources for each situation it encounters.

Questions for Discussion

1. Do you think healthcare professionals are realistic when they describe the characteristics of an IHT?

2. What methods might you use to get team members to open up about what the components and variables are for their team (i.e., which variables do team members exhibit and which variables are missing from the team)?

3. What phase of team development are you in and what phase is your team in?

4. What examples can you provide of complex common and complex uncommon problems, related either to patients or to your team?

6

Leadership and Power on Interprofessional Healthcare Teams

BOX 6.1 THE LEADERSHIP ROLE OF TEACHING

On a consulting trip I visited a healthcare facility where the medical residents made weekly patient rounds on assigned patient units. Most of the time the residents made rounds alone. When I met with them they groaned when I suggested they make rounds with the team members. I reminded the residents they were the most highly trained providers in the facility, and they had a lot to offer the team members in teaching them about the patients' medical problems. I then reminded the residents they didn't know the patients very well because they only saw them once a week. I told the residents they had a lot to learn from the team members who saw the patients every day and could brief them on potentially significant changes in the patients' behaviors.

Every member of the team must be able to teach and have a willingness to learn, because new problems will continue to arise. In their basic training few providers are schooled in the intricacies of teamwork. Many providers, including many RNs, have only a few years of formal training. They are trained to perform procedures but may not have the basic formal knowledge to think through unusual occurrences. The willingness to seek out learning experiences and to teach both team members and patients is a critical leadership skill for every team member.

In Chapter 2, we presented snapshots of the Westside Clinic team as it was going through major changes in the year 2000 and again in 2016. In both scenarios, the team physician was viewed as the leader of the team. In 2000, the nurse and social worker considered assuming leadership roles when the clinic was threatened. However, in 2016 it seemed as though the team members accepted the authoritarian leadership of the managed care organization as fact.

We can speculate about who the real leaders were in these two cases. However, it is more interesting to consider who should have been the leaders. The physician appeared to be the team leader because the administrator had communicated with him as team representative. The physician also seemed to have a lot of influence with the team, because in 2000, when he suggested the team accept the administrator's decision and stop meeting to discuss difficult cases, many of the team members appeared to comply. Perhaps the nurse practitioner and social worker would have exercised interprofessional leadership if they had gone to the administrator. However, if other team members did not accept the nurse practitioner and social worker in that role, their leadership would have been much less certain. And why, in 2016, did some team members seem more resigned to the decisions by the COO to decrease times for patient visits, while other team members resigned from the team? It is not clear if any team members other than the physician understood the difference in competencies between a social worker with a bachelor's degree (BSW) and one with a master's degree (MSW). It is not clear if any team member formally objected to the refusal of a social work position for the core team, or the decision to hire a BSW for the secondary team. It is also unclear if there is any ongoing dialogue between the members of the team and the COO. What is clear is none of the team members seemed to assume leadership to meet the needs of the clinic and the patients.

Thus far, we have seen that IHTs provide a forum for healthcare providers to address complex issues in patient care. Complex problems have many causes and effects that are initially unknown. Uncovering and addressing these related issues takes different kinds of leadership assumed by those who have the skills to define and address the underlying problems. Volumes have been written about leadership, and yet its essence remains largely misunderstood. We understand interprofessional leadership even less, as it has been researched very little. In fact, there is no widely accepted term for the kind of leadership that will be discussed in this chapter. Interprofessional leadership must take place in a way that allows health professionals to work across disciplinary boundaries.

Interprofessional leadership can be formal, informal, or both. However, the concept of interprofessional leadership is complex, and, even when it is understood, it may not be allowed or encouraged.

Background for Interprofessional Leadership

Organizational models and metaphors have influenced and will continue to shape the way that leadership is viewed in business organizations.[1] These models and metaphors refer to structural, behavioral, political, and cultural processes and are increasingly defining leadership in healthcare organizations in general and IHTs in particular, as more healthcare organizations are led by those trained in schools of management. Structural and behavioral characteristics are dominant in these models and metaphors.

Some of these models and metaphors are more favorable to interprofessional leadership than others. Structural models contend that leadership roles and functions in organizations are assigned and deliberate and that power is unevenly distributed.[2] An opposing behaviorist or humanist view suggests that the equalization of power in organizations is essential[3] and that shared leadership is basic to modern organizational development.[4] Leadership under the humanist tenets has been called unstructured, shared, informal, functional, empowering, participative management, consultative supervision, and joint consultation. Thus, the humanist view is much more consistent with what we have come to know as interprofessional leadership.

Despite the tension between these two models, most organizational literature focuses on both a technical and a human aspect. However, the human aspect of management is usually directed toward increased job satisfaction for the purpose of decreasing turnover and increasing production. And, despite the fact that structural and behaviorist models are each viewed as useful, the machine/structural model of organizations was paramount during much of the twentieth century.[5]

Models and Metaphors for Interprofessional Leadership

Leadership on IHTs in the early days of healthcare teams (1940–1975) was highly influenced by the field of group dynamics.[6] That influence was both positive and negative. While on the one hand it allowed time for tending to team process issues (e.g., encouraging every member to speak up and be heard), on the other hand it did not allow enough time to establish dynamic structures that would encourage efficiency of team operation.

Development of IHTs in the late 20th century was more influenced by organizational theory and by the structural models and metaphors that have been most prominent in organizational theory. Katz and Kahn stated that "every act of influence on a matter of organizational relevance is in some degree an act of leadership."[7] However, they referred to the leadership function as directed by the formal leader. In fact, it is very difficult for organizations to give up the concept of one formal leader. And although this concept should be synergistic with informal or interprofessional leadership, organizations tend to ignore the informal in favor of support for formal leaders.

Although most IHTs exist as part of larger organizations, they are not necessarily synchronous with them. If you ask healthcare professionals why they chose health care as a field, most will admit that it was because they wanted to help people, solve difficult healthcare problems, or be in a prestigious field. They probably would not say that it was because they wanted to lead a team. The desire to lead is uttered more often by those who chose management for a profession. In management circles, interprofessional team leadership is usually not thought of at all or is considered a management phenomenon. In fact, it might be difficult for managers to share the leadership function with those who aren't managers, because legitimate authority in bureaucracies has traditionally been accepted only through formal hierarchical structures. Recognition of informal leadership would contradict the basic purpose for which managers were trained.[8] This situation is a primary reason why interprofessional leadership has not been widely accepted.

Given the organizational focus on hierarchical structures and formal leadership, it is interesting to speculate what models of organization those who are involved with IHTs use. One study[9] reviewed the proceedings from the Interprofessional Healthcare Team Conferences (1976–1985) to see if the authors advocated that teams and their leaders take on particular strategies for dealing with conflict. The author categorized the papers using the four organizational frames proposed by Bolman and Deal,[10] that is, *structural* (achieve goals); *human resource* (serve human needs); *political* (use coalitions with different values); and *symbolic* (see organizational events as important for what they represent). The author found 21 of 180 articles referring to conflict. The papers advocated the human resources frame (16/21 or 76 percent); the structural frame (4/21 or 19 percent); the political frame (3/21 or 14 percent); and the symbolic frame (3/21 or 14 percent). More than one frame was advocated (6/21 or 28 percent). The structural and political frames (to be used alone) were each advocated only once. The symbolic frame was never advocated alone and was always coupled with the human resource frame. The author speculated that the recommendation for use of the human resources frame might reflect the historical basis of IHTs (i.e., small group and group dynamics theory).

At a workshop for healthcare and health administration professionals, the trainer introduced Bolman and Deal's four frames by asking the participants (N=31) which frame was primarily used by their hospital directorship and which frame was used by their immediate team. The responders were healthcare providers and administrators. Fifty-two percent thought the structural frame was the primary management strategy used by the hospital *and* their immediate team. Thirty-nine percent thought that the political frame was the primary strategy used in their hospital, and 32 percent thought the human resource strategy was the primary strategy used in their team. The remaining participants were uncertain which strategies either the hospital or their team was using.[11]

These case studies are centered on the leadership function of addressing conflict. In reflecting on these case studies, the concern is the discordance between how healthcare workers think they behave, their perceptions of how they think their organizations behave, and the perceptions of those who write about IHTs. Espousing only one or two models is not conducive to rapid change. Having access to many models of IHT and leadership is useful for developing IHTs that will survive within our changing times.

A third case study[12] revealed that interprofessional leadership is far down the list when health professionals think of IHTs. However, there is evidence that healthcare professionals adopt many models and metaphors about leadership and teams. These metaphors may be different from those carried by professionals who are not in health care. Healthcare professionals who were members of IHTs were asked to list the metaphors that came to their minds when they thought of healthcare teams. They generated metaphors that were grouped into 15 themes. The most commonly cited theme was *chaos/conflict* (e.g., "never ending battle, ram treatment down people's throats, dumping ground"). *Dynamic organism* was the second most commonly cited category (e.g., "plant, anthill, geese flying south"). The category of *leadership* (e.g., "collection of egos looking to Billy Martin for leadership, mountain-large base with stacked leadership and physician at top, eight horse chariot—who's in charge and where are we going") was sixth in order of citations. All but two of the ten metaphors listed in the leadership category were negative. Of those that were positive, only one, "soccer—balance of power and importance," reflected interprofessional leadership. The machine metaphor (e.g., "well-oiled machine, engine being overhauled by high school shop class, large machine with integrated functional parts"), which would fit with the structural models, was eighth in order of citations. The large diversity in metaphors cited speaks to the complexity and diversity of interprofessional healthcare practice. It also highlights the needs of health professionals for training in interprofessional leadership.

Leadership Theories

Although management is not the same as leadership, many individuals interchange these two concepts. The exercise of leadership by managers is characterized by the ability to reward and punish and also by the power of legitimacy.[13] Managers and administrators are designated as formal leaders. However, leadership that is exercised by those who are not formal leaders is more nebulous. Healthcare providers who are not formal leaders also have access to many powers of leadership, including rewards (nonmonetary), punishments (usually covert), and legitimacy (knowledge/expertise). Some group researchers define nonmanagerial or informal leadership as an outcome of leadership.[14, 15] Schön acknowledged that the role of leader can and does exist without the burdens of management, and managers are not necessarily leaders. He treated leadership and management as one and suggested that anyone can perform the symbolic, inspirational, educational, and normative leadership roles that he classified as the art forms of management.[16]

Returning to the case in Chapter 2, we find the nurse and the social worker in 2000 ready to defend the need for a team to the clinic administrator, who wants them to stop their weekly team meetings. The clinic physician, who was designated by the clinic as the team's formal leader, does not plan to take any action to counter the administrator's decision. He wants to accept the decision of the administrator and get on with patient care. In fact, the case does not state who is the formal leader of the clinic team. Perhaps the team has no formal leader. More likely, it is considered to be either the administrator or the physician. Perhaps the nurse and social worker should have ignored the unspoken rules and assumed a leadership role in this situation. It might have been the only way to save the team in the clinic. Or, they might have lost their jobs. The team was reenergized in 2016; however, it appeared that not much had changed in regard to team leadership.

Because leadership as it is applied to healthcare teams emanates from the organizational literature on leadership, it is important to understand a little about organizational leadership theories. At least six categories of leadership theories have gained popularity during the past 100 years. Three of these categories constitute the earlier theories of leadership and focus mainly on "the" leader.

Early Leadership Theories

Early leadership theories focus on the person in the leadership role. *Trait Theories*,[17, 18] a group of early theories, propose that leaders have certain characteristics that can be measured and, like intelligence, are probably inherited. *Behavioral Style Theories*[19, 20, 21] propose that there are simple linkages between leader style and effectiveness, and also that there is a taxonomy of leadership behavior. *Contingency Theories*[22, 23, 24, 25] combine the style and trait theories with situations in the environment that require specific approaches to leadership.

Later Leadership Theories

The later leadership theories focus on the culture of an organization and are characterized by *Exchange Theories*,[26, 27] where leader emergence depends on the possession of certain traits, and on group tasks and norms for skills and values that the group finds rewarding. Anyone who exhibits competence in the group's tasks and conformity to the group's norms can emerge as a leader.[28, 29] *Cognitive Theories* include Attribution Theory,[30] which implies that it is knowledge of outcome that determines our imparting qualities to the leader, rather than the conventional view that it is our experience of leadership that determines outcome.[31] Cognitive models might involve scripts that are played out by organizational members,[32, 33] and person schemas where workers automatically assess traits of leaders by matching their characteristics or behavior with personal perceptions of what leaders should be like.[34] *Transformational Theories* focus on establishing a goal or vision, the concept of change, and the involvement of followers in that change. Transformational leaders empower followers to act.[35, 36, 37] Other authors contend that in all of the cultural theories, leadership interrelates with the context from which it arises.[38]

It is clear that the later group of theories is more consistent with the type of leadership that is most useful on IHTs. However, organizations seem to be reluctant to accept and support interprofessional leadership. Healthcare organizations, despite the high levels of educated staff, are no exception. In fact, despite the large number of publications on teams during the 1990s, organizations appeared to be returning to earlier theories where leadership is focused on one leader. However, as the 21st century dawned, teams in general took a new interest in action learning, where teams evaluate problems in real time and team members assume leadership to make corrections.[39] Some surgical teams have developed action learning as a way to improve patient safety. Although attempts are being made to teach healthcare trainees and practitioners to assume leadership roles, what happens in the classroom and in workshops does not always translate well into practice. Leadership as an interprofessional phenomenon is still in its infancy.

Hollander, who noted that multiple leader roles could coexist in groups, set the stage for informal leadership in groups.[40] Others viewed leadership as both a property of a group and a process of human communication[41, 42] and concluded that leadership is neither the person in a formally established position nor any one person performing in the role of leader. Jago also defined the process of leadership as "the use of non-coercive influence to direct and coordinate the activities of the members of an organized group toward the accomplishment of group objectives. As a property, leadership is the set of qualities or characteristics attributed to those who are perceived to successfully employ such influence."[43] This definition fits IHTs because it does not restrict the leader to one who is formally appointed by the team, and yet it allows for addressing complexity and ambiguity. Also, leadership is seen as a dynamic process where leaders and followers exchange roles.

Essential Elements of Interprofessional Leadership

Rather than viewing interprofessional leadership as qualities in one person, it might be more appropriate to think of it as a system (see Figure 6.1) in which the behaviors of all team members play a role. Interprofessional leadership involves at least six elements: (1) environment, (2) situation, (3) leader(s), (4) team members (followers/peers), (5) power, and (6) communication. Like interprofessional teams, the elements that comprise interprofessional leadership are complex and changing. The effectiveness of the leadership will depend on the team's ability to see readily what leadership elements need to be in place in any given situation.

Environment

The team environment refers to everything (internal and external) that creates the backdrop for the team, for example, social structure, rules, physical setting, organization of work, structures for communication, history, team culture, politics of the organization, phase of member

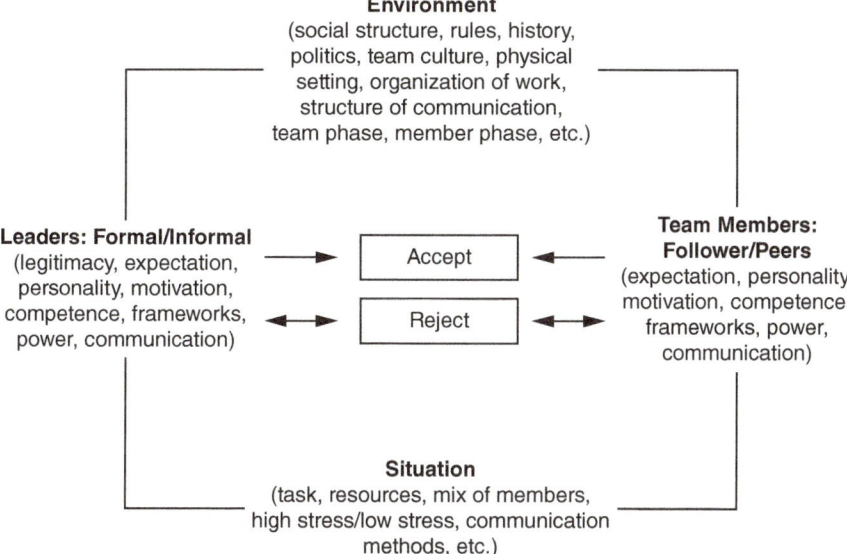

Figure 6.1 **Essential Elements of Interprofessional Leadership**

development, and phase of team development. Social structure, organization of work, and structures for communication fit together to create the framework that helps decide what kind(s) of formal leader(s) are needed for the team. However, that decision can be tempered by the politics of the larger organization.

It is common for the administrators of a healthcare organization to appoint formal team leaders who are not able to support the needs of a team. It is also common for teams to organize in ways that do not support the leaders they appoint. For example, if you set up a monthly meeting with the administrative representative for the health system and the leaders of the team at a time when the formal leader of the team cannot attend, it will create problems. You will get less done, you will have to double check facts, and it will be less efficient. While this sounds like an obvious problem, it is a frequent occurrence in IHTs. In some cases, the physician is established as a formal team leader but is not involved in key administrative discussions with representatives of the healthcare system. Conversely, in cases like long-term care facility teams, the physician "leader" might not have time or not wish to be involved in team discussions of clinical issues. In such cases, it is very difficult for the physician to represent the needs of the team to the larger organization, without defined structures and procedures for ascertaining the team's needs.

BOX 6.2　A CHANGING TEAM CULTURE

In one situation, an IHT had formed with many young members, and they began socializing once a week after work. As increased patient loads contracted their formal meeting time, some team business was conducted during the social hour. Gradually the makeup of the team changed, as did its culture. Team members were slightly older, with young families, and some of them were unable to come to the social hour after work. The ratio of females to males increased, and the few males on the team no longer came to socialize. Some team business was still conducted during the social hour, leaving members in both the old and new cultures wondering how rules had changed without them being aware of it.

If some team members socialize outside the work setting, the team's culture may partially be formed without the awareness of other team members. The team's culture also might change with long-term or part-time team members being unaware of that change. The team needs to review regularly its culture and identify changes as they occur.

The rules to which the team subscribes can be stated or unstated, made by the organization and/or the team, and rigid or flexible. Usually, it is not the rules that are inflexible; instead, it is the unquestioned way they are interpreted and accepted that makes them rigid. When team members interpret rules as guides to help them accomplish their mission, they realize that the rules need periodic reevaluation, especially if the majority of current team members did not invent them.

Environmental factors, such as structures for communication, are extremely important, and teams should review them and make their rules for using them explicit. This is particularly important as newer technologies for communication emerge. If the organization initiates a team, but does not allow for structures and resources to support that team, the team will likely not perform as well as it should and will probably not survive. Organizations that don't want teams, but somehow feel compelled to initiate them, will frequently not assign resources to support them. If an organization sets up a "virtual team" (where members do not work from the same location) without allocating computer networks, mobile

---

BOX 6.3   WHO IS RESPONSIBLE?

A group of professionals who worked together in a clinic called themselves a team, but they had never met as a team because the clinic in which they worked had no place that was convenient and available for them to meet. The team blamed the organization. The organization didn't understand the problem.

---

phones, apps, computer hardware, and processes for communication, the team is set to fail. In many cases, an organization will initially allocate these resources when the team is formed, but may not support the rapidly changing technology. The hardware slows down or malfunctions; the signal is blocked and communication suffers.

The ways that the team environment influences leadership are limitless and should play a prime role in reviewing leadership on the team. Most of these environmental factors are malleable. However, they need to be recognized before effective changes can be made. Both team and organization have a responsibility to recognize forces in the environment that will be detrimental to the team.

Situation

The situation is another major variable for interprofessional leadership and refers to the task(s) at hand that requires the team's attention. Situations that call for leadership have qualities of simplicity and complexity, normality and abnormality, straightforwardness and ambiguity, and high and low stress. The qualities of the situation should dictate which team member(s) lead and which ones follow. A situation might have little complexity, low ambiguity, and low stress and have too many members attempting leadership of the situation. In that case, members will be stepping on each other's toes and getting in each other's way. Another situation might be extremely complex with high ambiguity and high stress, and attract one or two team members who are not trained to take on the work for which the task calls. If the environment is such that structures have been put in place for such a circumstance and the team members have been trained on an approach, they will know the protocol and know which leader to call on if the need arises.

Leaders (Formal and Informal)

Interprofessional leadership encompasses the complexity of the tasks that are before the team and the immediate and long-term resources that should be applied to those tasks. Each team situation that calls for leadership will involve leaders (formal and/or informal) and team members (followers or peers).

Leading involves communication (ability to give and receive information) that is necessary for the team's work. Formal leaders are given a designated title by the organization or the team and are the types of leaders most often referred to in the organizational literature. Informal leaders can be defined as *anyone who moves the work of the team forward*. Team members can be formal and/or informal leaders or nonleaders if they refuse to assume any leadership. Schön was one of the few organizational theorists to acknowledge that the role of leader can and does exist without the burdens of management and that managers are not necessarily leaders.[44] This brings us to a realization that members of healthcare teams frequently have, which is that their formal leader is not the person they are following. Healthcare organizations don't always appoint the most appropriate team member as a formal leader. Such appointments may be based on hierarchy of discipline and do not give sufficient consideration to the appointed leader's knowledge of leadership tasks or the time the leader can devote to such a role. Some IHTs might be better off with several formal and/or informal leaders, preferably from different disciplines. It is also important that formal leaders be assigned to the team for sufficient amounts of time to perform their assigned leadership roles.

Team Members (Followers/Peers)

It has been said that leaders manage meanings.[45] In this regard, team leaders interpret team events and the climate in which the events take place. However, there can be no leaders without individuals who are willing to follow. Followers provide a context or background that invites a leader to lead. Otherwise, the leader will be seen as ineffective and will not succeed. Leadership involves considerable trust, as followers accept some form of symbolic power from the leader. Because trust is such a major issue in IHTs, the accomplishment of leadership tasks is much more important than having one charismatic leader.

Some theorists view participation as the influence that comes from someone being active in decision making.[46] Expressing that influence is what followers do. There are few books written about followers, though

---

BOX 6.4   WHERE IS THE LEADER?

A middle-aged female physician worked on a hospital team as well as a long-term care facility team, and as she traveled between the institutions she was sometimes late for meetings. Although there were issues to be dealt with that did not involve the physician, the team would never start without her even when she was a half-hour late. When questioned as to why they didn't start the meeting without the physician, one nurse revealed the team had agreed the physician would be the meeting leader.

---

followers are as much a part of leadership as leaders. Followers are those who are not actively assuming leadership roles and yet have the role of accepting or rejecting leadership. All members of the team are followers at some points in time, and thus all need to know how to follow. Like leading, following involves communication as the ability to give and receive information. Followers are continually assessing whether those who are leading are performing the necessary tasks of leaders; whether they as followers are adhering to the team's mission; and whether there is a gap in leadership that they have the skills to fill. The example in Box 6.4, above, speaks to the responsibility of followers in interprofessional leadership.

Power

Leaders and followers alike need to feel a sense of power and to understand their ability to contribute to the team's development and maintenance. While there are many power sources available to team members, some sources of power have a greater potential to add value and strength to the team. Evidence suggests that leadership is related to social power because observers confer it and the functions of leadership as a social influence process are shared throughout a group.[47] Other researchers see power in organizations as shared and deriving from activities rather than individuals.[48] Thus, the power in organizations is not static, because it stems from the context of the situation, and situations are constantly changing. This fluid notion of power is similar to that of influence, defined as getting results through social interaction.[49] Social influence can also be defined as leadership.

A study of a geriatrics team found that commitment, professional knowledge of geriatrics and/or team, energy, and organizational skills, that is, the ability to organize to solve a problem, were the major sources of power in a developed IHT.[50] Those members who had all four sources appeared to have more power within the team. Additional sources of power included tenure with the team and dedication to improving geriatrics and/or team. Personal attributes like charisma appeared to be important power sources in the early phase of a team's development. However, as the team grew, these personal attributes became much less important. In a subsequent study, Drinka found that the ability and willingness to teach and learn were additional sources of power for interprofessional leadership.[51] Thus, members who enter a developed IHT having knowledge, commitment, and personal and professional values consistent with the needs of the patients to be served will likely assume power for leadership on the team. They should also assimilate into a developed team more quickly than members who have knowledge and values that are inconsistent with the patient's needs.

Communication

The need for appropriate communication, or the exchange of information between team members, is the element that is integral to each of the other elements. Each team member has a responsibility to ensure his or her communications are being received and understood by the other team members. Both leaders and followers must be aware of the environment and the situations the team must confront, because they likely will need to switch roles depending on the environment and/or the situation.

Charismatic leaders have a natural ability to determine the social milieu of a situation and to shape that milieu to fit their needs. However, charismatic leaders may not play a large role in developed IHTs. It is likely that the more substantial power sources like commitment, knowledge, organizational skills, and the ability to teach and learn will be more powerful for demonstrating leadership, at least on developed IHTs.

The Interprofessional Leadership System in Action

Tasks

If interprofessional leadership is really a system of interactions, it is probably not accurate to think of leadership roles. It is more accurate to think of tasks of leadership. Rather than one role of "leader," an IHT has multiple leadership tasks and a multitude of opportunities to assume such tasks. Some of the tasks of interprofessional leadership are seen in Table 6.1. A member might perform many, if not all, of these tasks at certain times. Some team members might perform few of these tasks. It is unlikely that a member would be able to perform all of them all of the time. In general, members of healthcare teams appear willing to perform certain leadership tasks and to ignore others. Teaching healthcare providers how to perform the tasks of interprofessional leadership should make them more willing to assume them.

Table 6.1   Important Interprofessional Leadership Tasks

Organizer/Mover	Finisher	Expert
• initiate team development • identify team tasks • identify strengths/weaknesses • call meetings • provide structure • review team needs • identify appropriate patients	• impose time constraints • focus on outputs (patients treated, goals achieved) • seek progress • show high commitment to task • manage projects	• have special expertise • offer professional viewpoint • identify complex problems for interprofessional input • use expertise of other disciplines • understand patient needs • know team's expertise and limits
Ambassador	**Diplomat**	**Supporter**
• build external relationships • promote awareness of the team's work • build bridges • show concern for external team environment	• build understanding between members • negotiate • mediate • facilitate decision making	• build team morale • put team members at ease • ensure job satisfaction • help patient work with team
Judge/Evaluator	**Process Analyzer**	**Facilitator**
• listen critically/seek truth • evaluate clinical process and outcomes • help team reflect • promote appropriate clinical treatment • act logically	• identify member conflicts • analyze team problems • consult with team members • offer observations • help members to define team problems and design solutions	• identify conflicts related to clinical care • help team members find ways to resolve conflicts • help implement solutions

(*Continued*)

Table 6.1   (*Continued*)

Creator	Innovator	Challenger
• generate new ideas • visualize new programs/ projects • visualize new alliances	• discover resources • identify opportunities • transform ideas to strategy • propose new methods	• offer skepticism • look in new ways • question accepted order
Team Reviewer	**Quality Controller**	**Conformer/Follower**
• observe and review team performance • promote review of structure • give feedback • review consequences of team structures	• check output alignment against team goals • inspire higher standards • assure team reviews clinical outcomes	• seek agreement/ cooperate • fill gaps in teamwork • help relationships • avoid challenges • maintain continuity
Guard	**Teacher**	**Learner**
• protect team from too much output • protect team from too much input	• help new members learn norms and values of the team • teach shared leadership skills to other members • recognize leadership potential • teach others when to seek specialty advice	• ask questions, to enhance understanding across disciplines or areas • question the need for interprofessional input

In times of high stress for the team, members will likely perform the leadership tasks that are most related to their primary area of training. The leadership task that health professionals feel most comfortable with is that of "expert" in their field. Some might also feel comfortable with the tasks of "finisher, supporter, diplomat, ambassador, organizer/mover, and conformer/follower." Other leadership tasks, such as process analyzer, facilitator, challenger, and team reviewer, are tasks that health professionals were not necessarily trained to do nor do they like doing them, especially not across disciplinary boundaries. Yet these latter tasks are critical for the survival of interprofessional teams. Unfortunately, they are usually not viewed as part of professional practice, which is the reason they are the first to be ignored when a team is under stress. Some healthcare professions like social work, psychology, and psychiatry receive more training in these latter areas. However, even members from these professions might choose not to assume these tasks when the team is under high stress.

There are systems that have made successful attempts at training and enabling physicians to engage in peer-to-peer counseling when the process analyzer, facilitator, and team reviewer roles are required. Vanderbilt University has developed a stepped up system where the first encounter by a volunteer peer counselor/leader mentions the maladaptive behavior to the team member engaging in it, hoping the team member will get the hint and stop the behavior. If the behavior continues, team members will begin collecting data on the incidence, background, and severity of the maladaptive behavior to try to discover potential causes for the behavior. The initial efforts are to make sure the system isn't promoting the behavior before the peer counselor turns to the physician for rectification.[52] Such an approach requires a system that is set up to train and support peer counselors who willingly take on the role of process analyzer and to back them up when that is necessary. Ideally, an IHT would develop to the point where team members could assume these roles across disciplinary boundaries.

Matching Leader to Type of Problem

When is it appropriate for team members to fill in or to cover for other members, and when is it not appropriate or dangerous to do so? To answer this question, you must take into account the different levels of professionals and paraprofessionals who might constitute the "team," the amount of time each has to devote to the team, and how much and what kind of training they have had in working on IHTs.

IHTs have tight staffing patterns and may be constructed and staffed with part- and full-time members. In many cases, the MD/NP/PA is assumed to be the team leader, even though the MD/NP/PA may be with the team the least amount of time of any team member. In this case, the appropriate assumption of leadership by another team member should be standard practice for the team. The following vignette demonstrates some ways team members assume leadership roles when an IHT is functioning well.

Agnes: "A team I worked with on one of the wards performed really well. Initially we had our team meetings once a week, and then we said that was not enough. The team included MDs, nurses, PT, OT, dietitian, and the social worker for that unit. We could get stuff done and things were moving great with our discharges and support services. We had it down to a science. I knew it worked well, because we were having JCAH visit and we were told a surveyor was coming to observe our team. It wasn't a day the team was scheduled to meet. I had to email everyone and I was expecting one physician, but all four docs showed up. The surveyor asked an MD if he was required to be there. He said, 'I wasn't required to be there, but

I was asked to be there and I am part of this team, and we work together.' No one looked at it as a burden. There was a combination of personalities. The docs rotated in there, but the tone was set and it continued because it was the expectation. People saw the value and thought this is how stuff gets done here. They tried to overcome the reputation of the team being slow, and realized they could be efficient and still give really good care to the patients. The social worker and I were the leaders. It was a dual thing and we would have to prepare. If I was not there, the social worker or another nurse would take over. Everyone knew which patients were going to be discussed, so they had to come prepared as well. People would speak up. Decisions were made jointly. Sometimes nursing had information that social work didn't have. The social worker knew all the patients, but not all the details, so she would get information from her nurses before she went in. The team would talk it over and, for example, sometimes social work would step in and say, 'You might feel a patient should go to a long-term care facility, but they don't want to.' Sometimes you would need to let people go home and fail. You couldn't be dogmatic, and you had to look at the whole picture, and the team helped you do that."

It is important that team members know when to assume leadership and when to accept leadership from others. It is helpful to think of leadership as a way to address team problems. Problems can range from simple to complex and from common to uncommon (see Table 6.2). A simple common problem is one that occurs frequently. It might have more than one solution. However, the solutions are not ambiguous. An example of such a problem is deciding who will perform the leadership tasks at the patient care conference. Any team member can take on leadership and, with proper training, can perform one or more of the leadership tasks required for a successful conference. However, the team should have rules that the team approves. This will help distribute the tasks and keep the informal leaders from wearing out.

Any team member should be able to alert the team or, with appropriate skills, solve an uncommon problem that is simple. This might involve a social worker reviewing a patient's medications or monitoring blood pressure on a home visit, or a nurse securing a ride to a clinic visit for a patient who missed his ride due to a bladder accident.

When problems are complex, any team member can take responsibility for alerting the team to the problem. However, if the problem is common, the team should designate a leader and usually establish some kind of practice guidelines, so the team can try out mechanisms for solving the problem and evaluating feedback from the results. An example of a

Table 6.2 **Leadership Responsibility for Different Types of Team Problems**

	Simple	Complex
Common	A. Anyone can solve problem. Need rules for response to keep informal leaders from wearing out. Informal/Formal leader	C. Anyone alerts team to problem. Team designates leader and establishes practice standards. Formal/Informal leader
Uncommon	B. Anyone can alert team or solve problem. No rules; even new members are expected to take responsibility. Informal/Formal leader	D. Anyone alerts team to problem. Formal leader leads or designates a leader. Formal/Informal leader

common complex problem is arriving at a format for writing interprofessional treatment plans. Interprofessional treatment plans do not focus on patient problems that are discipline specific. Instead, they see the patient as a whole individual, with subsets of interrelated problems and interrelated solutions. Agreeing on a format for writing interprofessional problems is a complex task that requires a strong and knowledgeable leader. Having a defined format for such a common problem will increase the efficiency of the team.

When the complex problem is also uncommon, a formal leader may want to take the lead or to designate a team member as leader. Expecting a primary care clinic to absorb another clinic's geriatric population would be an example of an uncommon complex problem. A formal leader is helpful in such situations because that individual has more legitimacy with the administrative side of the organization. Also, since it takes time to solve complex problems, assigning a leader legitimates the application of that team member's time for a specific purpose.

Why Interprofessional Leadership Is Difficult

Training in autonomous function is central to the training of healthcare professionals. Discipline-specific leadership is focused on exhibiting skills in one professional area. Healthcare professionals are trained to think critically about their profession's segment of a complex problem. This is the way that most schools of health professions have been structured. Perhaps this is because this makes it easier for educators in those schools to ensure that "the core body of knowledge" for their discipline is maintained. Interprofessional education is complicated and somewhat messy. Our educational institutions are not structured to encourage cross-departmental teaching, because it involves a potential loss of resources. Also, cross-departmental evaluation often involves a perceived loss of control.

The training of other healthcare providers is primarily technical (e.g., clinic assistants, nursing assistants, licensed practical nurses, associate degree nurses, diet and pharmacy technicians, and activity, occupational, and physical therapy assistants). These individuals receive anywhere from six weeks to two years of training. Because of the technical nature of their training and the fact that they have to learn so many methodologies in a short time, they learn to accomplish the routine procedures they are expected to perform on a daily basis. In other words, they learn to deal with simple common problems.

Clinicians with more training or more experience will learn to deal not only with common simple problems, but also with "their part" of a common complex problem. They will not define a complex problem as complex, because that would suggest they might have to deal with other disciplines to solve it. They will also see solutions as certain because to imagine the ambiguity would threaten their identity as a practitioner in a specific field. Instead, they are taught to see a portion of a complex problem as *their* problem, in effect making a complex problem simple so they can address it. There is no time to learn the type of interprofessional thought processes that must go into framing and solving uncommon complex problems, especially problems that are also ambiguous. There is no time to learn about the complex decision making that can create a true resolution to such an issue.

The next step is critical for understanding why interprofessional leadership is difficult to assume and to develop. When healthcare workers encounter crises, as they do on a daily basis, it leads to stress. As healthcare professionals mature, they may learn what other professions are about and what to expect from different levels of workers in those professions. They might learn to work with many different disciplines on multiple levels. However, this situation changes when they become stressed. Stresses for health professionals don't just come from patients; they also come from other things in their environment, for example, conflicts with other workers, family problems, too much work, not enough direction, changing healthcare regulations, changing leadership, and changing ownership of their institution. When the environment for healthcare workers is very stressful, they revert to working the way they were trained to work, because it reduces their personal stress. They tend to lose sight of the need to work with members of other disciplines or even with other levels of their own discipline. They retreat into an autonomous mode of operation, because that is what is comfortable.

These comments are not meant to fault the thinking of paraprofessionals. They are intended merely to point out that, because of the training these practitioners receive, they are limited in the scope of their practice. The problem emanates from the payment structures that are allowed in some healthcare situations, the making of regulations, and the clinical translation of those regulations. Focusing primarily on financial issues, healthcare institutions often hire the least skilled worker that is mandated to perform a job. They tend to divide up health care into tasks that need to be performed, rather than the health that needs to be tuned up, regulated, or restored to an individual. Administrators might not be too bothered by the loss of seasoned clinicians, because those vacancies enable them to hire new healthcare graduates at lower salaries. These short-term strategies to save money upset the balance of leadership on IHTs. Loss of team members or key allies within the system is a reason for the IHT to reexamine its leadership structure and processes.

Assuming Interprofessional Leadership: Evidence for Why

Despite the fact that most healthcare professionals receive leadership training related to their profession, there is evidence that some healthcare professionals can and do learn to assume interprofessional leadership. This evidence shows what conditions lead a health professional to assume this type of leadership. I conducted a case study of leadership on a well-established IHT.[53] This section addresses some of the results of that study. All of the quotations from providers are from that study.

It is helpful to review the essential elements of interprofessional leadership (see Figure 6.1). In my study, the leadership *environment* on the team that was studied was a culture of valuing ideas, and the team atmosphere was one of teaching and learning. Study participants repeatedly mentioned this culture of valuing. Participants also noted that the *situation* had to be one in which they felt secure enough to assume leadership. Followers watched for models and mentors within the team. They admitted learning from them and developing a readiness for when they felt safe enough to assume leadership. Members who took on leadership often had prior experience as leader of a team. Mostly they would take on leadership because they felt secure in doing so. None of this is surprising, except that interprofessional leadership appears to be a set of skills that is separate from other professional skills that members had learned. It was also different from other leadership skills that most had learned.

The merging of a team's expectations for a member to take on leadership and that team member's readiness for assuming leadership are separate but related forces that affect the leadership practices on the team. A member's state of readiness may not match the state of the team's readiness for that member to assume a leadership task. Some members appear ready to assume leadership on joining the team. Others (even well-seasoned clinicians) might feel they are not ready and hold back for months, if not years. Some members might be ready for leadership in areas such as clinical, but not evaluation or process/relationship, counseling. The team's expectations of a member may prompt some *reluctant leaders* to take on a role for which they do not feel ready. Other members who do not feel ready may stand firm in rejecting an invitation to assume a leadership role.

Prior Experience and/or Training

Prior experience and/or training may be a factor in why some health professionals appear willing to assume interprofessional leadership, even when they are new to an established team. It appears to be part of the cognitive map they have for themselves. A member's readiness for assuming interprofessional leadership tasks in a clinical area was most often expressed as a feeling that their experience had prepared them to be a leader in their field. This related to readily assuming difficult clinical roles on the team.

BOX 6.5   INTERPROFESSIONAL LEADERSHIP RELATED TO PRIOR EXPERIENCE AND TRAINING

"From childhood on I had always been told that I was capable, and I had the expectation that I can always do what I set my mind to. I've never viewed myself as a star. I wasn't a straight A student. I wasn't scholarship material, but I always was told that I was capable. So certain expectations were set out for me, and I always had the feeling that I could achieve." *Nurse*

"I think it is partly because I knew what I was getting into when I got here—unlike some other fellows [physicians]. Because I had done the elective and had spent a month on home care and knew that it was a team approach. And I knew a little bit about what the dynamics were. And so I was very comfortable with the approach." *Internist*

"I think I had a pretty good background. Coming from the university for 10 years and floating through all of the services there doing some teaming over there. Yes I was ready and I think I knew enough medicine to feel comfortable going into the homes and I certainly have learned a lot of medicine from the docs in particular. I had done acute care, intensive care, and the burn unit, so sick people don't bother me. Frail people don't bother me." *Physical therapist*

Natural Leaders

The concept of having *natural leaders* on healthcare teams appears to be alive and well. When healthcare professionals encounter someone that they perceive to be a natural leader, they automatically have expectations that the person will assume some leadership tasks on the team. An administrative assistant remembered observing the team and choosing people that she thought would be *natural leaders* in certain areas. She also felt that other team members did the same thing. One team member had an interesting concept about team leaders. He felt that you could learn to provide leadership on a team but that you had to be a *natural leader* in order to lead when the team was having difficulties.

Box 6.6   Interprofessional Leadership Related to Natural Leaders

"And others saw it in that individual and it sort of evolves because, that person, it's apparent that they are a leader and then it just evolved and that person took it on and others encouraged it." *Administrative assistant*

"I took on leadership because I think that's my nature. I need to be able to express that. That time (when I was on the team), I was expressing that through my work." *Pharmacist*

"With my friends they always naturally looked to me as somebody who has good advice, who has some wisdom, and that I am able to problem solve. So I think it is something that I have always done. I don't think it is something that I had to learn to do. I think it is something where you learn about different people and different personalities, and learn how you can work with them and have a common goal and be able to make change." *Nurse*

"Until that social worker came on board, I think there wasn't a sense of leadership and I think that it was easy for the support staff to see that this new member was the person to deal with, because it just seemed like it was a natural leadership role for that person." *Administrative assistant*

"When the team works well, having inherent leadership qualities is less important. Then those non-natural leaders really blossom, because they are able to take and run with ideas. I think that during those down times those who actually did the leading would be those who were the natural leaders, who had tough hides, and who tended not to care in the long run that someone thought it was a bad idea, but would take and go with it anyway against the odds. I think that even in those circumstances, even though that person might be influential and might have a good idea, because of the nature of the team things got done very slowly if at all." *Pharmacist*

Reluctant Leaders

Although teams might have expectations that certain members should assume leadership, those *chosen* members might not be ready to assume the leadership tasks that others expect of them. Sometimes chosen members will take on the tasks in spite of their not feeling ready. Other times they won't. Some teams might be more tolerant of a member's refusal to assume leadership tasks. Other teams might not ask again even if the member felt ready at a later time. Some team members might never feel ready to take on interprofessional leadership. Some team members' views of leadership were more likely related to their discipline-specific role on the team and not to interprofessional leadership.

BOX 6.7   COMMENTS FROM RELUCTANT LEADERS

"If somebody expects you to do something, you just do it whether you like it or not. You were brought up that way too. You don't bitch, you just do it, and then you do the stuff you like to do later." *Physician who assumed a leadership role without feeling ready*

"I got involved to do what I thought was a better job for myself in relation to the patient, to do more of what was expected of me and to fulfill my role better. I just simply didn't have time to worry about the team as a functioning team. I only had time to worry about my relationship to the patient and my relationship to the team as far as the role that I was supposed to do. And that generally took more than my job time." *Physical therapist who refused to take on a leadership role that was expected*

Now You See Them, Now You Don't

Some members might become involved in assuming leadership on the team and then, for personal or professional reasons, withdraw to a less intense level of involvement. This may be temporary (e.g., when a member returns to school for extra training or goes on maternity leave). For some members, an initial withdrawal from leadership tasks may be the beginning of a permanent withdrawal process from the team (e.g., a member is mandated to increase time spent elsewhere or decides to take another job). Although the team might tolerate periodic withdrawal by a member with special expertise, it might result in that member not being viewed as an interprofessional leader by some team members. The withdrawal from leadership may be particularly difficult for some, as they will be perceived as less powerful during the time of their absence and subsequently upon their return to the team.

BOX 6.8 THOUGHTS ON BEING A SOMETIME LEADER

"The social workers were very good at teaching me boundaries at saying no. I used to think, give me everything. I can do it. But I learned that people will not think less of you just because you say no, I'm at my limit I can't do it. That was a big thing I learned on the team. I remember the feeling of control and reduction of stress I felt when I was given a golden opportunity to participate in this big thing and it was my choice to at this time say no. And before that I would have felt I had to do it." *Nurse*

"Leaving the team left a void." *Pharmacist*

"I missed the team so much, that professional interaction and the quality of specific team members." *Physical therapist*

> "I have to be able to retreat, and to do what I want to do when
> I need to do it. And if I am too directly involved in some activities,
> then retreat becomes difficult because I feel I bear a larger part of
> the responsibility. I don't mind being responsible for certain things,
> but I have to limit that exposure because it risks then that I do other
> activities less well." *Physician*

Additional clues as to why team members do or do not assume leadership might be found in some of the metaphorical themes generated in the study I coauthored.[54] "Resentment of the physician as leader (absentee landlord)" might prompt a "natural leader" to fill in the leadership gap, especially if they are a longer-term team member. Looking at leaders as "a bunch of unfriendly quarterbacks" might keep a potential leader from assuming leadership tasks and risk being identified with that group. A "stalemate" metaphor might also keep potential leaders from assuming leadership in a team culture where everyone is waiting for someone else to make the first move.

It is important that IHTs not close the door on any member's potential for leadership. For some individuals it might take more time, more training, or simply more professional maturity for them to be willing to assume leadership. Some team members may never be ready. It would be helpful to make the expectation for interprofessional leadership explicit in the primary training that professionals receive.

Assuming Interprofessional Leadership: Evidence for When and How

Strong Feelings

The *when* and *how* members assume leadership tasks are tied together and difficult to separate. Also, a range of variables regulates when and how members assume leadership. Themes from my study[55] included strong feelings about an idea or a situation; expectations by self and others; and development of a commitment or a common trust between the team and the member who was targeted for leadership. The major triggers for involvement in a leadership role included a sense of enthusiasm/excitement about an idea/issue or a sense of frustration/anger about a situation. Combined with the excitement, there was considerable evidence that team members recognized the added work responsibility accompanying the assumption of leadership as a trade-off for self-defined job satisfaction.

Associated factors included length of experience in clinical practice, availability of formal leadership roles in the team, and percentage of time the member is assigned to the team. Some members choose to get involved early in their tenure, while others spend several years observing the team to assess the nature of their future leadership role and/or a leadership role for another member of the team.

Box 6.9 Excitement as a Stimulus for Assuming Interprofessional Leadership

"I took on a leadership role because I felt very strongly about some of the issues that were coming up, and so I felt like if I wanted to make changes that I thought were important that I should get involved." *Physician*

"We did it because it was exciting. It was a challenge, and there was fun about the team being a bastard outside of two big bureaucracies, and to this day we carry the stigma and resentment of some people, because of that attitude that we manifested and the way in which we operated but we also achieved. And nothing is perfect, so I guess I don't know that we have to be." *Nurse*

"It was just so exciting. And then we wanted to let everyone else know about it because it was this great thing and we were doing this great stuff." *Social worker*

"It feels good if you can make an impact and change things to make them better for the patient as well as staff satisfaction." *Nurse*

"I was learning something new and I love to learn. I have memories of some very high energy discussions in the hall with people, things that we were excited about and thought we ought to be able to investigate, things that we could do to grow. So I guess just in terms of generating ideas, I think that it wasn't so much my role in doing that, but that I had a need to do that. That was part of what made it stimulating, to stand around with team members and talk about what we could do if we had the resources." *Psychiatrist*

"I did have an interest in being involved in something that was innovative. That was enough motivation there to be involved in that." *Occupational therapist*

"That's a buzz. When you get a roll going with this stuff it is just a kick." *Occupational therapist*

"I find it gratifying to work alongside other people on projects, having them appreciate ideas that I come up with and being able to work with them on those ideas." *Psychiatrist*

"In almost all instances there was a payback to me personally in that being able to motivate this group of people. There was an incredible amount of support aside from actually joining in and helping to get the job done, it was sort of the recognition of the accomplishments and the completion of the task. That you could really feel good about it without having to worry if it was in your area of specialty or not. Both of those made it incredibly easy. Also, it was an incredible learning process." *Pharmacist*

BOX 6.10   FRUSTRATION AS A STIMULUS FOR ASSUMING INTERPROFESSIONAL LEADERSHIP

"I changed the policy because it was something that I felt so strongly was a waste of time." *Physician*

"I was motivated, because it was a problem that was dissatisfying either to myself or to others as well." *Administrative assistant*

"I was angry. I mean I felt that the system was basically designed so the patient could always call the same audiologist, social worker, or whatever, but I felt the patients were not getting good medical care. It was so haphazard in how it was being performed. I felt the physicians were always being usurped, basically by the team members, to the detriment of good patient care." *Physician*

"Because I had some expertise in that area or an interest in it. I got involved with the treatment plans because the ones we did initially I considered just busy work. You wrote on them, and you never touched them again until two months when you had to write on a separate sheet of paper, re-write all your goals and all of your objectives. I thought that was a waste of time that I didn't have." *Nurse*

"Just the fact that you are a doctor you are legally and morally responsible for the patient. If it is directly associated with a patient, you have to facilitate it and if you don't you are a mess." *Physician*

"I do have an idea of what is correct almost all of the time. Even if things aren't black and white, there is a better way for most things, to initiate therapy or treat a patient. So you get involved to get it done the best way, and maybe prevent a lot of the big time problems." *Pharmacist*

"If we did something a little different, we could either anticipate what was going to happen to the patient or provide them more or better service." *Physician*

"I get involved, because if you don't get involved when you see a change coming or you see the need for change, you don't have any say in what happens. Things change around you and you are totally out of control." *Social worker*

"Some of the things that would come up at times were sort of disruptive, and it felt like they were undermining things that were there and were o.k. But there was a lot of it that I could agree with, when it resonated with my own sense of feeling repressed. That was sort of a prompt for a more productive discussion for how we could change things. And so I think some of the less idealistic, I have to make my job better, kind of complaining was another factor." *Psychiatrist*

"I can remember lots of times the hallway discussions we would have were bitch sessions, and I think that kind of complaining sometimes also generated new ideas and impetus for change." *Psychiatrist*

Some tasks of leadership that are appropriate during one phase of a team's development are not necessarily those that will work at another phase of a team's development. Also, since team members may be at different phases of development, a particular task of leadership may be more relevant for some than for others. There is no way that one designated team leader could be expected to perform all of the tasks of interprofessional leadership that an IHT needs to grow and maintain itself.

Team Members' Perceptions of Leaders

Each team member can usually identify the formal team leaders. Team members seem less certain about who the informal leaders are in a particular situation. Healthcare providers who are seen as informal leaders by their teammates may be reluctant to view themselves as leaders. I studied the development of leadership and the perceptions of team members in an IHT that had evolved over a period of 15 years, with no assigned internal leaders and with little direct formal leadership.[56] This study focused on whether or not formal and informal leadership developed within the team, how leaders developed, and what made team members assume leadership roles.

Table 6.3 Selected Characteristics of All Team Members during a Nine-Year Period

Profession/ Discipline*	Gender	A-Self Perception (%)	B-Others Perception (%)	Difference A–B (%)	Years on Team	Time Devoted to Team (%)	Formal Leadership Role
RN	F	100	98	+2	>3	100	Y
MD	F	100	91	+9	>3	V*	Y
SW	F	100	91	+9	>3	V	Y
PSY	M	100	89	+11	=3	V	N
SW	F	100	85	+15	>3	100	Y
MD	F	0	75	–75	<3	V	Y
OT	F	0	75	–75	<3	50	N
PT	F	83	74	+09	>3	25	N
AA	F	0	74	–74	>3	100	Y
MD	M	100	66	+44	>3	V	Y
RN	F	71	63	+08	>3	100	Y
SW	F	—	63	—	<3	V	Y
SW	M	0	58	–58	<3	100	N
RN	F	75	57	+18	>3	V	Y
PH	M	100	55	+45	>3	V	N
SW	F	—	55	—	>3	100	Y
MD	M	—	55	—	<3	V	N
RN	F	—	53	—	<3	50	Y
RN	F	—	53	—	<3	50	Y
RN	F	0	53	–53	>3	V	Y
PT	F	0	50	–50	<3	V	N
MD	M	100	47	+53	>3	V	Y
PT	F	0	44	–44	<3	50	N
PH	F	40	44	–04	>3	40	N

MD	M	0	43	–43	=3	V	N
RN	M	0	42	–42	<3	100	Y
MD	F	0	42	–42	<3	V	N
PSY	M	100	40	+60	=3	V	N
OT	F	0	39	–39	<3	50	N
OT	F	—	36	—	>3	V	N
MD	M	—	36	—	<3	V	Y
RN	F	0	36	–36	<3	50	Y
MD	F	0	35	–35	<3	V	N
MD	M	100	32	+68	<3	V	N
RN	F	50	31	+19	<3	V	Y
MD	M	—	29	—	<3	V	N
RD	F	—	26	—	<3	50	N
RD	F	—	25	—	<3	50	N
MD	F	0	22	–22	<3	V	N
OT	F	—	21	—	<3	50	N
PSY	M	—	21	—	<3	V	N
OT	F	0	20	–20	<3	50	N
PT	F	0	19	–19	>3	V	N
MD	M	0	16	–16	<3	V	N
MD	F	50	14	+36	<3	V	N
MD	F	—	14	—	<3	V	N
PH	M	0	10	–10	<3	40	N
RD	F	—	07	—	<3	50	N
MD	M	—	06	—	<3	V	N

* V=Variable; RN=nurse; MD=physician; SW=social worker; PSY=psychiatrist; OT=occupational therapist; PT=physical therapist; AA=administrative assistant; PH=pharmacist; RD=dietitian

Thirty-four team members were asked to identify the members of the team who were leaders during each time period that they (the interviewees) were members of the team. Over a span of eight years, there were nine separate time periods representing intervals of stable team membership. Data on (A) a member's perception of self and (B) others' perception of a member are compared in Table 6.3. This table lists data by professional discipline, gender, percentage of time an individual rated self as leader out of the number of times possible, percentage of time an individual was rated by other members as a leader of the number of times possible, the direction and percentage of the difference, years on team, percentage of time on the team or whether that percentage varied, and whether a member had a formal administrative role on the team.

Self-Perceptions of Being a Team Leader

There was variety in the team members who perceived themselves as leaders of this IHT. Team tenure appeared to be a major factor in establishing a self-perception of interprofessional leadership. Members with longer tenure generally had stronger perceptions of themselves as leaders than those with shorter tenure. However, neither discipline nor gender of members seemed to be a factor in whether or not members perceived themselves as leaders or in their perception of the consistency of their leadership over the years that they were a member of this team. It was no surprise that those who had formal leadership roles were more apt to perceive themselves as leaders than those who did not.

Team Members' Perceptions of Others as Team Leaders

Data from Table 6.3 on members' perception of others as team leaders revealed that members differed in terms of who and how many members in a given time period they perceived as leaders. Members did not necessarily view the same members as leaders in all time periods that they were on the team. Some team members did not list other members as leaders during time periods when those members demonstrated physical or emotional absences from the team. It is clear that team tenure did play a role in that longer tenure tended to increase the chance of a member being perceived as a leader. Also, formal leadership role seemed to be associated with being perceived by others as a leader. However, a formal leadership role did not guarantee that others would perceive a member as a team leader, especially if those being rated were transient members of the team. No member of this team was rated as a leader 100 percent of the time. This situation indicates that even the highest rated leaders were not always matching some members' perceptions of leadership. The members who at times did not perceive the team's needs for leadership as being met, even by the highest rated leaders, tended to be those who were themselves perceived by others as leaders.

As the data in this study were compared it became clear that several other factors ensured members would be perceived as leaders. Members who were seen as either extremely competent clinicians or as extremely creative problem solvers were seen consistently as leaders. Finally, when members appropriately assumed the leadership task of "process analyzer," it ensured them of being perceived by others as powerful leaders on this team, whether or not they had a formal leadership role.

Team members who were not perceived by others as team leaders tended to be newer members (less than three years) of the team. The one factor that almost guaranteed members would not be perceived as leaders was whether or not they had been forced to join the team or felt like they had no other choice. There were times when administrators would assign someone in their department—often someone who was seen as a misfit in his or her department—to the team. If joining the team was something that a clinician did not want to do, it made it difficult for that person to assimilate into the team and almost impossible for that individual to assume any interprofessional leadership tasks.

Large Differences in Self-Perception and Others' Perceptions of Team Leaders

Perceptions of leaders varied by team member. Each member appeared to have a perception of who the leaders were for any given time period of team membership. These attributions or cognitive schemas pertained to both the member's perception of self as leader and the member's perception of other team members as leaders. All members of the team had a discrepancy between the percentage of time they perceived themselves as

Table 6.4   Members with Greater Than 19 Percent Discrepancy between Self-Perception and Others' Perception of Leader

	Overestimate	Underestimate
Males	5	3
Females	1	12

N=21 of 11 males and 23 females who performed the exercise.

leader and the percentage of time others perceived them as leader. However, some members had a large discrepancy (>19 percent) between how they rated themselves and how others rated them as leader. There was greater than 19 percent discrepancy for 21 (8/11 males and 13/23 females) of the 34 members who performed this exercise. Gender appeared to be a variable in either greatly overestimating (male) or greatly underestimating (female) one's self-perception of leadership. The trait of physician was also associated with greatly overestimating one's self as leader on the team. And male physicians seemed to be the most prone to believing that they were exhibiting team leadership when in fact they were not, or at least it was not being recognized as such by the team. Another study described those who overestimate their authority as naive group members and noted that those individuals usually characterized themselves as natural leaders.[57]

Administrators often expect physicians to assume the role of formal leader. Despite this expectation of leadership, physicians often have limited leadership training and heavy time commitments. While physicians expect to assume leadership on IHTs, they might not be the most appropriate healthcare professional to assume a role like team coordinator. Also, the nature of a patient's perceived problems might dictate the assumption of the leadership role of care coordinator by team members who are not physicians. The high status of the profession of medicine establishes the strength of this double bind.

The female leaders in my case study[58] appeared unsure of their informal leadership potential and the impact of their informal leadership on the team. Since this is a case study it is not possible to extrapolate to female members of other healthcare teams. However, it is possible that females tend to greatly underestimate their potential as leaders of healthcare teams. Also, little team longevity and low percentage of time on the team cannot be underestimated as factors in creating faulty perceptions of leadership.

We need to think of mechanisms that will close this gap between the perceptions and realities of leadership, especially if we are talking about healthcare professionals job sharing, working on multiple teams, or making virtual teams work. IHTs are complex social systems that exist within other complex social systems. As such, we should expect that the leadership of IHTs would be a complex phenomenon. Rather than thinking that we can identify certain traits of leaders, it may be more helpful to identify situations in which leadership should play a role, and members are expected to assume leadership tasks. The concept of singular leader should be abandoned since no one leader can provide all the leadership in any complex situation. Instead, we might think of opportunities for leadership in a leadership system.

Additional Leadership Responsibilities

Patients and Team

Although the patient's role in the team has been addressed in articles on teamwork, this is a controversial area that has not been well defined. Like team members, patients must at times assume the tasks of leader and follower. Although patients are not core members of the team, they are at the core of what the team decides and the work it does. The capacities of patients to participate in their care differ markedly. The very nature of being a patient means that you need someone with more knowledge about certain areas of health care. This need puts patients at a perceived power disadvantage and perhaps it is why they are often reluctant leaders as in the following vignette.

BOX 6.11 PATIENT AS RELUCTANT LEADER AND UNWILLING FOLLOWER

Marty: "I am a relatively healthy young male who is depressed and have been seeing my primary care doctor for treatment. I just got a call from Dr. B's nurse about my blood level and it was very high. However, she remembered that I had asked if time of day mattered (the time the blood was drawn). So she began asking around (Dr. B is out of town), and no one on the team seemed to know anything. Apparently there are supposed to be at least 12 hours between taking the drug and the blood draw. At best there was a 10-hour difference. I can't imagine that it will make a big difference since the reading was so high, but, I will go back and let them draw again tomorrow morning. The high level might explain the tremors I have been having in my arms and hands. I asked another physician who I know and she said that this medication has a long half-life (time it takes the level of medicine to drop in half) and that two hours wouldn't make any difference in the blood level. I am not sure why they waited to do a blood level, probably a cost-saving measure that enters into their evaluation at the end of the year. First I was too low, then I got pushed to an appropriate level and was doing fine, so instead of leaving the dosage alone Dr. B increased it hoping that would move things along more quickly. I called him a few days after I started taking the higher dose to tell him that I didn't feel well, but he just said he would wait to get a level when I returned for my regular appointment. Now I am at too high a level and am having all kinds of problems. I am thinking of finding another physician, but

---

> I have been going to Dr. B for so long and I don't know who might be good. I would like to decrease the dose, but I don't want to do it without his permission. Next week when Dr. B is back I am going to encourage him to refer me to a psychiatrist."

What began as a relatively simple and common case had the potential to become complex. To avoid that probability it required communication and a team effort between the nurse, the internist, a psychiatrist, and Marty. That did not happen soon enough, and Marty was hospitalized. This case reflects the ambiguity that many patients feel when they know something is wrong, but they don't know how to engage the team in a way that will ensure them the best care. It is not clear who has the responsibility to teach patients how to participate in their care and how to most effectively interact with the team. Currently the popular press attempts to teach patients how to interact with their physician. However, this is a complex topic, and little is done to address the patient's relationship to the team.

The team and the organization housing the team have an obligation to see that the patient knows the team's members, what they are trained to do, how they work together to provide care, and what their options are if they feel they are not getting the care they need. The patient has an obligation to keep track of treatment effects and to be honest and open with the team. The team has the daunting task of learning what kind of care the patient and family want and integrating that knowledge with their expertise at providing care. This is a dynamic process that requires good communication between the patient and team systems.

Administrators and the Team

Administrators have an obligation to be interprofessional leaders as they provide vision and resources for the team to perform its work. They are also expected to be followers by observing and evaluating the team's work and attending to areas where they can help the team to succeed. They must listen to the needs of the patients through the collective eyes of the team and translate that knowledge into the ever-changing world of healthcare financing.

Leaders Need the Power to Lead

Amy: "I am a nurse supervisor for ten teams that care for adults with chronic and acute physical and mental disorders. I received a verbal message from a nurse that one of the patients on her team had requested a transfer to another team. The patient was in the process of contacting other teams in the organization. The team members had decided they had tried everything they knew to help this patient, and he continually rejected their treatments and attempted to manipulate the team members by telling one of them one thing and another team member something else. A week went by and the patient decided he did not want to be transferred to another team. The team decided to proceed with the transfer anyway because all of the team's members were exhausted by this patient and thought another team might be able to take a fresh approach to the man's care.

I alerted the COO to the situation because I felt this patient would likely go to the press with a story of being wronged by his healthcare system. The COO chided me for not helping the distressed team deal with this situation and gave me a lecture on how to treat patients. I felt dishonored and proceeded to tell the COO that he had his head in the sky and simply didn't understand what those in the trenches were going through. I suggested all top administrators should attend some team meetings, go with clinical staff on home visits, and attend clinic visits so they have a better idea of reality."

In addition to management respecting the concerns of clinicians, different levels of management must learn to respect one another. Repeated disrespect of this nature often reflects the culture within the broader organization. If the top leaders of an organization do not structure a system that supports its leaders at all levels, it will not be able to support the development and long-term survival of IHTs.

Summary

This chapter began with the definition of interprofessional leadership as moving the work of the team forward. As we end the chapter we would like to present a revised definition.

BOX 6.12 INTERPROFESSIONAL LEADERSHIP REVISED DEFINITION

Interprofessional leadership is a systemic structure and process of:

- promoting relationships,
- moving the work of the team forward,
- directing the practice of health care toward the needs of the patient and the viability of the system, and
- using uncommon sense in common situations.

Questions for Discussion

1. What kinds of leadership exist on your team?
2. What kinds of leadership are missing from your team?
3. What kinds of leadership are most important for the kind of teamwork you practice?
4. What kinds of training have you had to help you assume team leadership?
5. What are your power sources?
6. What power sources do your teammates see in you?
7. If your team's physician came to work and you could smell alcohol on her breath, who on your team would address the problem and how?

7

Conflict and Problem Solving on Interprofessional Healthcare Teams

Conflict involves desires that are incompatible.[1] When healthcare providers from multiple professions and different levels of training are assembled in a team and expected to function, we would anticipate that there would be conflict. Unfortunately, just mentioning the word "conflict" elicits fear in many healthcare providers. Perhaps this fear stems from the discomfort that comes from knowing conflict can impede the progress of work and place us further behind. Or, perhaps it is that healthcare providers see themselves as helpers to people in need. If you see conflict as primarily negative, it seems out of place in a helping situation. Conflict just doesn't seem compatible with our image of a well-functioning IHT.

Conflicts within groups and organizations have been the subject of books and articles for many years.[2, 3] Articles about interprofessional conflict among healthcare providers or between healthcare team members and patients or between IHTs and administrators have been relatively scarce. More recently, there have been articles about conflict within medical action teams[4] and surgical teams.[5] Conflict does exist in all of these venues, and that conflict comes in many variations.

Conflict in work groups has been divided into three areas: relational, task, and process conflict.[6] Relational conflict is revealed when there is strain between group members that might be expressed as anger, annoyance, exasperation, irascibility, or somehow devaluing another member.

Task conflict relates to group members having different ideas over whether a task needs to be performed or the type of task. Process conflict relates to differences in opinions on how to perform a task. Although it is a general view that healthcare teams should focus on task conflict, all types of conflict exist on IHTs, even on high-performing ones. If there is more relational conflict than there is task or process conflict, it is a good indicator the team is in an early phase of development.

Conflict relating to team members might be obvious and open, but more often it is veiled by the cloak of the life-saving activities in which we busy ourselves. In the past, most interprofessional healthcare team literature was concerned with reducing conflict.[7, 8] Few articles have addressed conflict as a positive force.[9] Although conflict can be either a positive or a negative force for an IHT, conflict management might be the process factor that is most necessary for both innovation and survival of IHTs.[10, 11]

Conflict can also be seen as an essential part of team function and maintenance because it is inextricably tied to innovation, evaluation, and effective problem solving. Methods for constructively confronting conflict allow team members to move a team beyond its basic group development tasks and to promote frequent reevaluation of its established norms, goals, procedures, and outcomes. Confronting complex problems almost always involves conflict. How a team frames the problems and decides to address the problems will determine the quality of its problem solving. The way a team addresses conflict also speaks to how well developed it is. Skills in conflict management and integrative problem solving are essential skills for all team members. They are particularly necessary for those who assume the leadership role of teaching teamwork to their fellow team members and others who come into contact with the team. Evidence of constructive confrontation of conflicts is an indicator of an IHT's readiness to model teamwork.[12]

Types of Team Conflict

Intrapersonal

In discussing conflict, it is helpful to determine who is feeling the effects of the conflict. When you feel the burning in the pit of your stomach that so often results from conflict, it is tempting to think that the whole world is at war. However, intrapersonal conflict may only exist within one individual. In fact, you might be the only one who is feeling negative effects from an experience with another team member. While "The Meeting" incident described in the next vignette may reflect bad behavior on the part of the team, this appears to be an intrapersonal conflict.

> **Jane:** "I was fairly new to the team. However, I had worked on other IHTs and felt comfortable expressing my viewpoint in the team's meetings. A team member objected strongly to something that I said in a team meeting. In unison, the whole team said, 'no, we don't want that.' I kept quiet for the rest of the meeting. I felt terrible and was sure the team did not like me. My stomach began to hurt and I was beginning to doubt why I took the job. Several days later I approached one of the team members to ask why everyone at the meeting was so vehemently opposed to my idea. The team member told me they had tried that idea within the past year and found it to be dangerous to patients. The team member assured me no one was upset, and they realized I wasn't involved in the problems the idea had created."

It is possible the team could harbor ill feelings about Jane for bringing up an issue about which they had negative memories. However, this did not appear to be the case. Intrapersonal conflict can affect the team. For example, if Jane were to act differently toward the team because of what she experienced in the meeting, this could turn into another kind of conflict. If a nurse comes, sleep-deprived, to work after a major argument with his spouse, the nurse's mood will likely affect his interactions with other team members and, in subtle ways, with patients. We like to think of ourselves as professionals who leave our personal problems at the door. However, we are only human. Since conflicts escalate so quickly they are seldom of one type. Many interpersonal and intrateam conflicts start as intrapersonal conflicts.

Interpersonal

Interpersonal conflict occurs between two individuals. In relation to IHTs, this type of conflict could be between two team members. It could also be between a team member and a healthcare practitioner who is either part of the same healthcare system or part of another healthcare system. Another type of interpersonal conflict could be between a team member and a patient or member of the patient's personal support system.

> **Sue:** "I had been referred for a magnetic resonance imaging (MRI) scan of my spine. Having had previous MRIs, I remembered they were loud. I kept telling myself I would remember to ask for a pillow under my knees and earplugs for my ears. In the interaction with the technician, I remembered

the pillow, but forgot to ask for earplugs. After the first set of pictures, the technician asked me how I was doing. I told him I was very uncomfortable because of the loud noise and asked if I could have earplugs. The technician told me that he would have to start over if he brought me out. After the procedure was completed the technician suggested that if I was bothered by noise I should have asked for earplugs before the procedure. I asked the technician why earplugs couldn't be placed on the table for the patient to decide. The technician said that was not feasible because in the last several months I was the only person who had asked for earplugs."

Tom: "I am a pharmacist and was making hospital rounds with the hospitalist who prescribed what I thought was an inappropriate medication for a patient. I suggested another drug to the physician. He didn't say anything and didn't change his mind. I later sent him several articles about the drug I recommended. After that he was very cool toward me, and the other clinicians on the unit seemed less willing to take my advice."

Although these stories represent interpersonal conflict, it is easy to see how they could expand to other forms of conflict. Sue might have written a letter of complaint to an administrator or might have chosen a different MRI provider. Tom seemed to be experiencing a cold shoulder from his teammates, indicating his encounter with the hospitalist might have become an intrateam conflict. Because of the speed with which healthcare providers often work, it is sometimes difficult to recognize and check interpersonal conflicts at an early stage. When interpersonal conflicts are not recognized, they can rapidly escalate to intrateam or interteam conflicts.

Intrateam

Intrateam conflict is conflict that may start out between two members and grow to involve either part of the team or the entire team. When team members begin taking sides against another group of team members, you know there is intrateam conflict. The entire team might also be pitted against one of its members, either viewing that member as the scapegoat or the team being viewed by that member as being deficient.

Hank: "I was a psychologist in an outpatient geriatric assessment team that was part of an academic teaching hospital and its healthcare system. Dr. James, a geriatrician who was director of the assessment program, was a prominent physician within this system and was well liked and respected by his peers. One thing that really bothered me was when he refused to reveal the diagnosis of dementia to patients and their close family members, because 'they weren't ready to receive the information.' This attitude was problematic when the patient was still driving, and during my interviews with the patient's spouse I discovered the patient's driving behavior had become risky.

Over time I came to realize the situation was more complicated because Dr. James liked being 'adored' by his patients. He did not like giving them bad news. Also, Dr. James was on the board of this proprietary hospital, and board members were very concerned about their position within the very competitive community-wide healthcare arena. They did not want to lose patients. In a conversation I had with Dr. James, he admitted concern about the clinic's ability to attract more referrals, and he reminded me our mission was 'to provide hope to patients and their families.' The other team members were as upset as I was about our inability to truly help demented patients and their caregivers. Although I enjoyed working in the clinic, I left the position because I felt I was in an unethical situation that I had no power to resolve."

Intrateam conflicts are often about professional values, where members of one profession view a situation differently from those of another profession. When intrateam conflicts form along disciplinary lines, it is a sure sign that the team and/or some of its members are in, or have reverted to,

---

7.1   UNPRODUCTIVE APPROACH TO INTRATEAM CONFLICT

A physician who worked as part of an IHT clinic team did not like the way the clinic functioned. He was constantly complaining that it was inefficient and not well organized. He decided that he would invite the physicians who worked in the clinic to meet him in a bar after hours. He wanted to get the physicians' input regarding a plan that he had developed for changing the clinic operation. After the physicians who met in the bar had approved the new clinic plan, the physician who started this process presented his plan to the clinic coordinator, who was a social worker. The social worker, though skeptical of the new plan, suggested that the recommendations be presented to the entire team for input. Since the other physicians in the clinic had already agreed to the plan, when it was formally presented to the team its adoption was assured. The revised plan did not help clinic efficiency and made the nonphysician members very unhappy. Within several months the plan began to fall apart and within a year all traces of it were gone from the clinic.

BOX 7.2   CREATIVE APPROACH TO INTRATEAM CONFLICT

A physician who worked on an IHT that delivered home care was disenchanted with the format of the interprofessional care plan. She openly complained to the team about how awkward it was to write in the current format and also that it was not easy to follow the patient's progress. The team challenged the physician to change the care plan. The physician took up the offer and asked for team members to work with her in developing a new prototype for the plan. Team members also suggested other members who they thought could contribute to restructuring the plan. The volunteers formed a subcommittee with the physician and developed a draft of a new format that they brought to the team for comments. The new format was adopted and became one of the most successful innovations of this team's history.

---

an early *norming* phase or even back to the *forming* phase of development. Intrateam conflict can occur over differences in values between two subcultures of the team. In addition to professional values, those subcultures might be grouped by values that spring from any similar quality (e.g., age, gender, having to miss time at work because of problems with child care, or distractions because of ill parents).

Intrateam conflicts can also generate creative dialogue between team members who have achieved the *confronting* or *performing* phases. The nature and openness of the conflict are indicators of whether the conflict is healthy or unhealthy. The openness of the problem may also be contingent on how the conflict is defined by different members of the team.

Interteam

Interteam conflicts are true system conflicts. They can occur within one system between an IHT and another part of the system, or between two different teams in separate systems. In an era of limited funding by health insurers and limited support by some agencies, it is common for patients to move between healthcare agencies or between clinics within the same agency. This can cause conflict between health providers who don't normally work together, as they are forced to communicate. This is conflict that we cannot afford to ignore.

June: "I was a social worker for a medical home care agency. Brad was a patient who lived alone. He had many chronic health problems, and had been treated by our team for several years. Brad's beloved dog died about the same time Brad developed throat cancer. One day the nurse made a home visit and found Brad wandering aimlessly in his backyard. She quickly realized that he was hypoxic and suspected the tumor in his throat was constricting his trachea. Brad was quickly rushed to the hospital where it was the policy for the inpatient team to assume a patient's care. Aside from a transfer note or discussion, the home care staff was discouraged from visiting a patient until discharge was imminent. Several days after admission the home care staff received word that Brad was agitated, was constantly pulling out his tracheostomy, and in a hypoxic state was ripping off his clothes. The inpatient nurses were upset because they were unable to communicate with him. Brad's living will stated that he wanted everything possible done for him. A speech pathologist was called in and tried to teach Brad how to communicate with a communication device. The physician came in and told Brad he would not live if he did not keep his breathing tube in. The social worker from the hospital called Brad's friends and minister. Brad refused to communicate with anyone and continued to pull out his tracheostomy tube and rip off his clothes.

On a hunch, I stopped by Brad's room, looked him in the eye, and said 'I know what you want.' I told Brad I knew he wanted to go home. Brad shook his head in the affirmative. I promised Brad if he would keep in his breathing tube for two days I would try to take him home for a visit. This time Brad remained intubated. The next few days were hectic as the home care team negotiated the trip home. The hospital team was opposed to the visit saying 'Brad would not return to the hospital.' On the third day after Brad left in his tracheostomy, three members of the home care team (nurse, physical therapist, and social worker) signed Brad out of the hospital against medical advice and took him home where his neighbors and minister met him. The minister held a prayer meeting and Brad's friends took him to each room of his home so he could say goodbye. When the home care staff returned three hours later Brad was ready to return to the hospital. Two days later Brad died peacefully in his sleep. The hospital team continued to express anger at members of the home care team."

Handing off cases to other teams, organizations, or family members is a major source of interteam conflict. If the two teams do not jointly define the problem, there will likely be conflict. In the case of Brad, the inpatient team wanted to give the patient the best care possible, and they defined the care as reducing hypoxia. The home care team was defining best care as increasing Brad's quality of life in his last days. If both teams had defined the problem together, there likely would have been less inter-team conflict and Brad might not have suffered as much as he did.

Sources of Team Conflict

We have discussed three areas and four types of team conflict. How-ever, there are many more sources of team conflict. Each of the compo-nents and variables in the IHT model that were presented in Chapter 5 (see Table 5.1) is a potential source of team conflict.

Components That Directly Influence Practice

Unique characteristics of each team member—such as level of flexibil-ity and openness, coupled with the values, strengths, and knowledge each member has in his or her profession—can be stimuli for team conflict or cohesion. For example, a nurse who grew up in a family that avoided con-frontation at all costs would be influenced by that background. If team members are not secure in their professional knowledge, they are likely to avoid conflict. On the other hand, being a risk taker can be a source of conflict on a team where the other members are very careful and proce-dure oriented. A recently trained professional can be a source of conflict on an IHT that has little turnover, and where the members have not learned how to mentor or learn from a new member. It is especially help-ful to consider the components that directly influence practice as sources of conflict whenever the team adds a new member.

Intrateam Components

Internal structure and process components of teams can all become sources of conflict. Structural issues, like physical placement of offices, can be a major source of conflict when team members are not near each other and have not established structures for informal interaction and communication. Internal process components like problem definition can be a source of team conflict when patient problems are identified as discipline-specific and charted according to actions by individual dis-ciplines. If a team doesn't agree on structures and processes for conflict management or for teaching new members, or if the structures and pro-cesses established for these components are ineffective, conflict will ensue. Intrateam components are likely sources of conflict when a team changes its mission, experiences turnover, or faces changes in technical aspects of communication.

Organizational Components

Any of the components that relate to the internal organization or to external organizations that affect the team can be a source for team conflict. If a healthcare organization establishes IHTs, and continues its discipline-specific methods of evaluation rather than team-specific methods, that will be a source of conflict for the teams. If state and national policies for reimbursement do not support the use of IHTs with patients whose needs are complex and ambivalent, there will be conflict. Healthcare providers will be stressed and the patients will be upset for not receiving care that addresses them as whole persons. The shifting nature of the healthcare business continues to be a major source of conflict for IHTs.

Components for Team Maintenance

An IHT must have a way of collectively identifying its accomplishments and needs. If an IHT does not regularly present its accomplishments and needs to the larger system, it will be a source of conflict. By their nature, organizations consider direct team costs and benefits. They tend to ignore indirect costs of *not* having a team and the indirect benefits teams create. When economies shrink, organizations often see IHTs as liabilities. This tendency can create uncertainty among professionals and ongoing team conflict. Team members can help this situation by understanding the value their team brings to the system and acting as teachers to the larger system. If the larger system does not have a forum for learning about the accomplishments and needs of a team, it will be a source of team conflict.

Not Realizing What You Don't Know

It can be a recipe for disaster when healthcare providers are sure they understand something they don't. This is a common source of team conflict in teams that use ad hoc or formal work group methods of problem solving. It is also a major source for conflict between members of an IHT and those who are not members—patient, family, or other teams—especially when patient handoffs occur.

Professional Autonomy and Fear of Making Mistakes

Two additional sources of team conflict are worth mentioning, because they universally apply to healthcare professionals. They are *professional autonomy* and *fear of making mistakes*. Both sources of team conflict are

---

Box 7.3   The Handoff

A family practitioner, the only member of her group who had been fellowship trained in geriatrics, had recruited older patients with complex and ambiguous problems into her clinic. She had also assembled a small IHT consisting of a nurse and social worker. For the first time in three years, the geriatrician decided to go out of town on vacation. She asked her physician colleagues if they felt comfortable covering for her while she was out of town for two weeks. The physicians laughed and one of them said, "Oh that won't be a problem, we'll expect a few calls about adjusting Digoxin doses." The geriatrician replied that they would be more likely to receive a call in the middle of the night from a distraught caregiver because her elderly mother who has Alzheimer's has been found wandering around in the snow. The physicians decided that they should further discuss the call procedures. Since the geriatrician had the physicians' attention, she also told them what they could expect from the team members who weren't physicians.

---

linked to the unique cultures taught by each health profession and the training each profession mandates to retain that culture. These aspects of training within each profession are reflected in the difficulties they experience with teamwork. The performance of an IHT is based on admitting that different disciplines are needed to effectively treat complex problems in a particular patient population. The team must ensure a common definition of a patient's problems and open communication between the disciplines to determine type and sequence of interventions. Since a team's growth is based on its ability to evaluate itself and to correct its mistakes, members of IHTs must respect the cultures of other team members and be willing to trust all team members to observe the team's work and give honest feedback.

We have stated that schools of the health professions generally train students to function autonomously. Their leadership training does not teach interprofessional leadership, but rather it trains professionals to lead their professional colleagues. When healthcare providers must teach or give feedback to team members from other disciplines, it crosses a boundary most were not trained to cross and creates uncertainty, fear, and intrapersonal conflict.

In addition, healthcare professionals are trained not to make mistakes. However, health care inherently addresses life-and-death issues for patients who are at risk from illnesses that might not be fully understood. Consequently, health care is fraught with mistakes. And, healthcare providers will admit to mistakes in private conversations with providers of their own kind. Physicians are taught to learn from mistakes in venues like "tissue conferences" or "peer review." However, this learning is meant for physicians and is generally not meant to be interprofessional. And while these learning venues are common in academic settings during training, they do not necessarily carry over to nonacademic practice situations. When they are offered, they are scheduled at hours that make it difficult for some providers to attend. If admitting mistakes to members of one's own profession is difficult; admitting mistakes across disciplinary boundaries is unimaginable for some professionals.

Relationship between Trust and Conflict

Trust, in its most basic form, is a belief that someone is going to do what they say they are going to do or what they are expected to do. Trust has also been defined as one person's willingness to be vulnerable to another.[13] The person who makes herself vulnerable makes a judgment that the other person will act in a predictable way.[14] Trust has elements of reliability, predictability, and fairness.[15] Trust may well be the most important element in well-functioning IHTs. Conflicts that occur in settings where there is high trust are more likely to benefit team outcomes. Dr. Goodman and I developed a technology to determine team function and discovered trust to be the central mechanism in a well-developed team system.[16]

Trust has both a cognitive and an affective dimension.[17] In IHTs, trust develops when team members become familiar with the skills and behaviors of each other. A team member cognitively learns about the competence and reliability of a team member to do a job. When that team member also exhibits openness to feedback and learning, and expresses concern for the patients and other team members, a deep level of trust can be established.

Interprofessional trust is established over a long period of time. Trust enables cooperation and is the foundation for sharing mistakes across disciplinary boundaries. IHTs can establish safe interprofessional venues to learn from their mistakes. Team trust also enables conflict to be constructive. When team members trust one another, they can use conflict to

---

BOX 7.4   PEER REVIEW

An IHT initiated a process of interprofessional peer review. Annually, each team member was to fill out a short written evaluation on every other team member. The intent was to give constructive feedback. After the first round of evaluations, the physicians in the clinic stopped the process, because they said that members from other professions did not have the knowledge to evaluate their work.

---

create positive change. However, there is a negative side to trust, in that a team can have too little or too much trust. If a team has too little trust, members will likely not raise questions when they should for fear of being seen as ignorant, inadequate, or obnoxious. When team members trust each other too much, they will not raise questions when they perceive a potential problem, because they are sure their teammates "could not make a mistake."

The organization that houses the team must build venues for sharing mistakes into their formulas for financing teams. Without such a mechanism, there will be little learning across disciplinary boundaries. The IHT will not be able to grow as a team, and its value of freely integrating knowledge in complex cases will be lost. At the highest level of trust, each team member could act for another in certain circumstances, understanding the limits of each discipline. This level of trust takes time and is why the practice of rotating team members to different teams and departments can undermine the trust within a team and cause intra- and interteam conflict.

In this case, many of the physicians were new members of the team. It is clear the physicians had not had enough time to develop the level of trust in the nonphysician members of this team that would be required to conduct this type of peer review.

Limited Time, Uncertainty, and Constant Change

The appropriateness and quality of team decisions will be based on members' abilities to problem solve in the context of conflict. The stresses of limited time, uncertainty, and constant change, coupled with a team's lack of training, will produce conflict. Such conflicts enhance health professionals' fear of relinquishing autonomy and admitting mistakes. Thus, it is imperative that team members feel comfortable in recognizing problems with patient care and in discussing these problems (including their mistakes) with their teammates. This requires that, early in its existence, the IHT establish acceptable mechanisms for interprofessional reviews of patient care and team function. If written peer review is unacceptable, then an open forum for voicing concerns is necessary. When a mechanism for review is not jointly defined and mutually understood, conflict will escalate, causing regression to an earlier phase of development.

Preferred Responses to Normal and Conflict Conditions by Professionals Who Work on IHTs

It is likely the healthcare field attracts professionals who have certain preferences for responding to conflict. A study that looked at motivational preferences categorized the responses of 516 health professionals and advanced-level trainees who worked or trained on interprofessional healthcare teams.[18] Respondents were asked their preferences for interacting with others when things were going well and again when they were in conflict with others. When responding, professionals were asked to think not just about home or work situations, but generally about how they liked to interact with others.

Of seven preferences, the predominant motivational style of respondents under normal conditions was altruistic/nurturing (43.80 percent). This high percentage would be expected among individuals who entered the healthcare field. Under conflict, the preferred style was to withdraw and act autonomously (56.40 percent). There was more variation in style preferences under normal than under conflict conditions (e.g., assertive, analytic, and flexible styles). This study also compared the conflict styles for one team over five time periods. During the two periods of highest team stress, approximately 70 percent of the team members chose the autonomous style as their preferred style in conflict situations. This preference for becoming autonomous when faced with conflict among those who enter the healthcare field can cause problems for team members who need to jointly address conflict in complex situations.

Five Approaches to Conflict Management

As much as we would like to think of ourselves as rational beings, our responses to team conflict will involve some kind of emotion, and that emotion will manifest itself in numerous ways, direct and indirect, verbal and nonverbal (see Table 7.1). These emotions are expressed in

Table 7.1   **How Team Members Express Emotions in Conflict Situations**

Direct–Verbal	Indirect–Verbal
• describe feelings (consistent with the core values and ground rules that the team has set) • focus only on one point • blame others • deny one's actions • overdefend a position	• raise or lower voice • raise unrelated points • change opinion when pressured • spread the guilt • verbally attack members over unrelated issues
Direct–Nonverbal	**Indirect–Nonverbal**
• withhold relevant information • exclude essential disciplines	• be silent • glare • laugh or grunt • sigh • obey with animosity • avoid eye contact • slouch or sit erect • fold or wave arms • tighten facial muscles • conceal emotions

conjunction with the various approaches we take when managing conflict. Using different terms, researchers have outlined five approaches to conflict management: (1) coercing/forcing, (2) avoiding/withdrawing, (3) compromising/negotiating, (4) accommodating/obliging, and (5) collaborating/integrating.[19, 20] A more recent study has used four approaches,[21] leaving out the accommodating/obliging. However, this approach has a unique place in health care, particularly in mental health teams, and it should be retained. The chosen approach for any particular conflict is driven by past experience, training, motivation, and habit.

The five approaches to conflict can also be thought of as avenues to problem solving. Productively using any one of the five approaches requires knowledge of the power requirements, desired outcomes, and appropriateness of an approach for a given situation (see Table 7.2). A major departure from previous work is *acknowledgment that in the process of collaborating on an IHT, power within the team is frequently not equal,* but every member must have power for decision making.[22] It is at the level of integrative problem solving that the power lies with the team. An increased level of IHT development and a greater depth of culture will allow team members to freely exercise each of the conflict/problem solving styles and channel individual styles toward a collaborative approach. As an IHT matures, it should become more proficient at selecting the conflict/problem solving approaches that are the most appropriate for a given situation.

Table 7.2 **Using Conflict to Promote Interprofessional Problem Solving**

Methods/ Strategies	Power	Conclusion	Use/Don't Use IF
Coerce-Force/ One defensive; one offensive; emphasize differences; judge and accuse.	Imbalance (real or perceived); attempt to retain imbalance.	One yields or standoff.	Emergency; unpopular issue, fixed resources, need decision/ Need support or long-term relationship.
Withdraw-Avoid/ One defensive; one offensive; emphasize differences.	Imbalance (real or perceived); attempt to retain imbalance or create new imbalance.	One yields or standoff.	Trivial issue; little power; nonrecurring problem; part of larger problem/ Serious issue; critical goals; recurring problem.
Negotiate-Compromise/ Bargain; hoard information.	Relatively equal; attempt to increase relative power.	Different factions agree to accept decision; all win and lose.	Mutually exclusive goals of moderate importance; balanced power; focused on roles/ Early in problem; need more information.
Accommodate-Oblige/ Share *all* information, clarify *all* disagreements; equalize input.	Relatively equal; attempt to further equalize power.	Overt agreement; covert disagreement common.	When wrong; need social credits; goals not critical; to promote member responsibility/ Issue important to team and relationships.
Collaborate-Integrate/ Openly present problems; use all power strategies; balance conflict and cooperation.	Universal and unequal; members free to get more power; however, team controls power for team decision making.	Comprehensive solution and reevaluation.	Critical needs and goals; ill-defined problem; need commitment/ No time; no trust.

What We Think We Do Might Differ from What We Do

When we ask healthcare providers to name the approaches to conflict they think are most commonly practiced by healthcare professionals, the answer is usually collaboration and accommodation. It doesn't help that most conflict style assessment instruments allow people to think that collaboration is their preferred style of conflict management. However, when using more sophisticated conflict management instruments like The Conflict Management Survey,[23] it becomes clear that the preferred styles of healthcare providers are avoiding and coercing. Coercing and avoiding behaviors that emanate from fear of making mistakes can impede open dialogue with other providers. In fact, coercing and avoiding are intertwined. Although many people think avoiding is passive, it is actually an active style of conflict management. A team member cannot coerce another member unless that other member is willing to avoid or withdraw. Also, if someone actively avoids a conflict situation long enough, the avoider becomes a coercive force. If conflict isn't addressed, it tends to escalate and erode the trust and commitment of team members.

As a way to cope with their intrapersonal and team conflicts, team members often become masters of avoidance. If healthcare professionals perceive that they do not have time or do not know the appropriate strategies for confronting and resolving conflict, they will avoid it. They are more apt to avoid it in the *forming* and *norming* phases of team development. Box 7.5 demonstrates some of the many avoidance mechanisms used by healthcare providers to address conflict. The use of avoidance as a primary coping style impairs the ability of the team to function creatively and efficiently. By virtue of their training, health professionals feel that conflict should be avoided. However, their habits, motivation, and past experience may change that avoidance to coercion.

**BOX 7.5   AVOIDANCE: THE TEAM'S FAVORITE CONFLICT
MANAGEMENT STYLE**

1. **Patients come first.** Ignoring the concerns of a coworker on the pretext that you need to attend to the needs of a client, all the while planning to avoid the coworker's concerns.
2. **Strong emotions (blowing smoke).** Someone begins yelling at you regarding mistakes that were made. This takes the heat off of them because they realize that they have contributed to the mistake.
3. **Intellectualization.** If you cite authoritative sources you can usually avoid the conflict of being questioned.

4. **Rationalization.** If a person doesn't want to constructively approach a conflict, they can always find an excellent (and very rational) reason not to do so.
5. **Negativism.** "Yes but," "that won't work," "we've tried that" are all expressions of negativism that put people off and keep them from offering what might be important suggestions to alleviate the conflict.
6. **Procrastination.** Focusing on things that are "more important" because you really don't want to deal with the conflict. "I know I have to deal with this, but the patients come first."
7. **Humor.** Using humor to divert the focus from the problem so the problem never gets addressed.
8. **Compulsivity.** Focusing more intensely on the task to get it "perfect." "Maybe if we just keep doing this and get it right the conflict will go away."
9. **Slowdown.** Doing the task very slowly so that you don't have to face the conflict. "I'll do this, but maybe if I work slowly they will forget about it."
10. **Bringing in food.** It is difficult to address a conflict toward you if you have just engaged in such a "kindness."
11. **Positivism.** "Of course we can do that," "we do that all the time," "we already do that" are avoidance responses when used as a way to keep people from improving the process.
12. **Sunshine club.** "I don't know what you are talking about; we don't have a problem" is an especially powerful avoidance response when it involves team members who are leaders.
13. **Sick in**. A team member does not show up for a meeting or team training because they claim to be sick.
14. **Half-truths.** Addressing the less-difficult parts of an issue to temporarily get the monkey off your back.
15. **Electronic messaging.** When you are upset, using electronic messaging as a way of communicating with a colleague while avoiding directly confronting a significant conflict or issue.
16. **Beepermania.** When electronic alerts control the individual and allow him to use it as an excuse for avoiding unpleasant situations; continuing to use electronic devices during meetings or using them in ways that aren't related to the team task.
17. **Do what I know best.** "I'll just do my own job and not make any waves." "What is going on around me is none of my business even if it is affecting the team."

18. **Robert's Rules of Order.** Using strict rules to avoid all conflict—even when it might be constructive.
19. **Too busy—no time.** Thinking that we are so important that we cannot take the time to resolve a conflict.
20. **It would upset the patient.** Using a patient as a shield to avoid conflict.
21. **River in Egypt.** Denial is very effective in assuring yourself that a conflict really does not exist when the evidence suggests otherwise.
22. **Anything could happen.** Using vague but seemingly serious personal medical conditions as a way to keep others from confronting you.

BOX 7.6   SUNSHINE CLUB

A team pharmacist approached the formal leaders of an IHT (a nurse and a physician) to suggest that there was a lot of conflict among team members because some had not been properly oriented and others resented that the newer members did not know how to work on a team. The formal leaders rejected the suggestion that the team was in conflict, saying that everything was fine and suggested that the pharmacist was a "negative" person. As more new team members became disgruntled and left the team, the pharmacist went to the administrator at the next higher organizational level to repeat what he had stated to the formal team leaders. The administrator said that he had heard nothing but good news about the team's function from the two leaders and suggested that there really was no problem.

Stress and conflict trigger creative accomplishments in IHTs. Conflict can be used as an impetus for the team to innovate and grow. However, if members are continually stifled or coerced in terms of their change efforts, then team members may try to serve their own self-interests by turning on other team members. It is helpful to look at the types of conflicts that are occurring and how they are being dealt with in order to understand how to make them productive.

We all have experienced behaviors of a clerk or a waitperson that is stressed. If we see the conditions of the stress or are somehow aware of them, it is much easier to accept a longer wait for service. However, when the clerk or waitperson is exceptionally friendly, smiles, and says things like, "I will be right with you" or "your order is on its way" and nothing happens for a reasonable length of time, it results in feelings of helpless frustration. It is equally frustrating when a team member uses a cheerful style to avoid some conflict that has occurred or is occurring. In effect, this person is denying the conflict and choosing the avoidance style of the "sunshine club." This behavior is particularly forceful when powerful team members engage in it. Situations like this are even more frustrating when they involve communications problems within a system in which a team is working.

Matching the Type of Conflict to the Problem-Solving Response

Conflict Strategies as an Indicator of Team Function

The methods that a team uses to address or avoid conflict can be a predictor of that team's ability to function. They can also be used as an indicator of the team's current phase of development. While conflict is present in all phases of a team's development—*forming, norming, confronting, performing*, and *leaving*—it is addressed differently in each phase.

In the *forming* phase, members are guarded and unsure of their purpose. Conflict cannot be readily seen because it is neither discussed nor addressed. In this phase, conflict can be caused by differences in members' expectations concerning why they are on the team, expectations and uncertainty about what each team member will do on the team, worries about fitting in, and concerns about not embarrassing one's self or profession. These conflicts are often intrapersonal conflicts, and are seldom discussed. Accommodation may be overused in this phase. Coercion may also be heavily used in the *forming* phase. It is easy for one member to coerce other members in this phase, because they are relatively quiet as they try to find their places on the team.

In the *norming* phase, members begin to recognize that they don't agree on the collective goals and purposes of the team. Scapegoating is a common behavior for a team that is in the *norming* phase of development. It is probably not unhealthy for teams to have scapegoats, as long as the scapegoats do not last for more than a few days. When a member remains the team's scapegoat, it exemplifies a deeper problem, and perhaps reveals a team that is stuck in this phase. By accepting the role of scapegoat, a team member might indicate that he is stuck in an early phase of team development, even though the team might have progressed to another phase.

In the *norming* phase, members develop an expectation for "equal power." Team members might want to rotate leadership tasks in order to avoid conflict and maintain "equal power." In this phase, the team adopts policies as mechanisms to *avoid* open conflict. One team that was stuck in the *norming* phase imposed *Robert's Rules of Order* on itself. These were used during patient care conferences and prevented the team from intuitively addressing the difficult issues that kept it from maturing. Addressing conflict in writing keeps the source of the conflict hidden. Members might address ongoing team conflicts with written policies and procedures, where negotiation will be cautiously used. Frustration would be expected to build in the advanced *norming* phase, with an increase in defensive communication. Members might try to *force* ideas on other members as they struggle to retain their "equal power." Other members will avoid confronting aggressive team members as a way of retaining their "equal power." As the team approaches the *confronting* phase, conflict will begin to erupt. This conflict may frighten some members, who withdraw to the overtly more comfortable *norming* phase.

In the *confronting* phase, there may be increased conflicts over values, leadership, equality, and commitment. Again, the methods team members use to confront each other in this phase are a measure of the team's development. If some members use coercion and others counter with avoidance, there will be confusion as to which members are being *coercive* and the result will be a regression of members back to the *norming* phase. When some members realize their power for constructive confrontation and use the opportunity to engage in problem solving behavior, interprofessional leaders begin to emerge. As more members assume appropriate leadership tasks, there will be a realization that member power is not equal. To use conflict to its fullest potential, all team members must begin to realize their unique potential for power that enables the assumption of interprofessional leadership. In this phase, the members need to focus on framing interprofessional problems in ways that promote the assumption of power by members who have the skills to contribute to the resolution of a specific problem.

This is an example of two members of a team that was functioning somewhere between *confronting* and *performing* in its development, when it was bombarded by some very unusual stresses. This unproductive confrontation accomplished nothing, because the two individuals involved were both using coercion, and the outcome was a stalemate. The physician

---

BOX 7.7 UNPRODUCTIVE CONFRONTATION

A well-developed IHT was under extreme pressure to produce—even while clinic administrators were reducing physician staff. Several years previously, one of the team members had left her position as a nurse on the team to become a part-time administrator and educator to this and other teams. While the position cuts were looming, one of the physicians approached the educator and in a condescending voice said, "What do you do anyway?" The physician wanted the former nurse to return to clinical nursing to take some of the burden off the team. Rather than discussing the source of the cutbacks or whether the physician's unspoken idea made any sense, the physician devalued the educator's work and made the position of educator seem worthless. The educator was caught off guard and became defensive. Nothing productive was accomplished.

---

and nurse educator could have accomplished a positive confrontation by jointly defining the interprofessional problem with all of its variables. They could have brought the issue to a subcommittee for the team or to a team process meeting. In defining the problem, the nurse educator and physician should have focused on what the clinic was expected to accomplish (e.g., whether the clinic had the right mix of disciplines, whether the procedures for seeing patients could be streamlined to save time and still deliver quality, and what else could be done to alter team stress). The nurse educator and physician likely regressed to a *norming* phase of development, and hopefully they returned to the *confronting* phase and were able to open this issue and turn it into a learning experience that was valuable for the team's growth. If the entire team had returned to the *norming* phase, nothing would have been accomplished, and the anger would have grown.

The IHT moves into the *performing* phase when there is consistent evidence of constructive confrontation among members. Individual members feel free to demonstrate their power in the process of integrating solutions to team problems. In the *performing* phase, members might assume advanced teaching roles and protect the rights of their fellow members to use power.[24] By establishing individual power as a norm, the team ensures that a few members do not assume all of the power on the team and that every member has power for decision making. *Performing* can be seen when the conflicts are directed more at program development and efficiency than at individual members. Also, the differences of each team member become an appreciated addition to the team. Members have discussed differences in values and trust each other enough to view conflicts as normal. Both the ongoing team members and the entire team might continue to recycle through different phases as they encounter new problems.

Repeated unproductive conflict propels some team members to leave the team. The conflict might come from within the team, an individual, or the organization. Sometimes leaving is contagious and more than one team member decides to leave. A team member from such a team drew a picture at a team workshop. She depicted her team as a graveyard with names of the exiting disciplines on the gravestones. Mass emigration from the team often results from unaddressed conflict and can propel the remaining team members into the *leaving* phase. An IHT that is stuck in this phase spends most of its energy on grieving, allowing little energy for interprofessional problem solving.

The team can usually avoid the problem of mass emigration of team members by addressing conflicts as they occur and not allowing them to escalate. It is especially difficult if team members leave because the team didn't value them or chose to ignore their input. Every team member should develop multiple sources of power to increase their chance of being valued by the team.

Relating Power Currencies to Conflict and Styles of Problem Solving

There are forms and uses of power that are important in the management of team conflict. Every team member has access to and is susceptible to the use of power currencies. Power currencies are tangible and intangible attributes that are valued by people. They are things like respect, information, morality, trust, influence, enthusiasm, ambition, assertiveness, skills, well-being, orderliness, efficiency, logic, integrity, warmth, friendliness, openness, flexibility, beauty, and wealth. They can be any attribute that an individual finds attractive. In fact, these are the things that motivate us. Advertisers focus on attributes that we value in order to sell things to us. In the process of communication, colleagues and teammates use power currencies to "get our attention." Power currencies can form the magnet that attracts us to a certain individual. We might be attracted to people because we value trustworthiness and see them as trustworthy. Healthcare professionals in general have strong affinities for the power currencies of respect, morality, knowledge, helpfulness, and integrity.

As the fire that warms also burns, power currencies can be used in both helpful and destructive ways. In fact, the same power currency can be used with any of the conflict/problem solving methods. For example, if you were the pharmacist on the team, and we wanted to coerce you by using the power currency of "respect," we could say, "We will lose all respect for you if you neglect to give the patient the pain medication that he or she needs." On the other hand, we could also choose to use any other problem-solving style with the same power currency of "respect." Using the collaboration/ integration style we might say, "We are concerned that the patient is truly suffering; we respect your knowledge of the patient and wonder how we can discuss possibilities for more effective pain control." When healthcare workers overvalue a certain power currency, others might use that currency in coercive or avoidant ways to sway the workers to a specific way of thinking. Although coercive and avoidant methods of problem solving sometimes have their place, they do not lead to creative solutions for difficult problems.

Even if a team member does not value a particular power currency, but knows that others overvalue it, that team member might use that currency in various ways to manipulate team members to his way of thinking. Since there is often a fine line between problem solving and manipulation, the main concern is that the team's culture, in the face of conflict, promotes both freedom to problem solve and freedom to dissent.

BOX 7.8   COERCION IN A TEAM MEETING

A pharmacist was upset because the team physician prescribed a particular antihypertensive drug. The pharmacist knew the team valued knowledge and accuracy and chose a team meeting to ask, "Why was this drug prescribed when it has such terrible effects on orthostatic hypotension?" The venue of the meeting and the pharmacist's tone and words were coercive. The team physician became defensive and retorted with more coercion. If the pharmacist had approached the physician alone or with another involved team member, they could have engaged in an ad hoc problem-solving session and solved a problem before it got out of hand. If the physician still refused or ignored the pharmacist's suggestion, it would signal another broader conflict that might be resolved by using a team mediator. If the issues that arose from those meetings were team issues, the matter could be brought to the team for discussion.

Addressing Ongoing Disruptive or Maladaptive Behavior on the Team

The term *disruptive behavior* was co-opted for use in health care to describe interactive human behaviors in health care that have the potential to disrupt care or create an unsafe environment.[25] These behaviors include being abusive, intimidating, demeaning, disrespectful, dishonest, undermining, and in violation of professional boundaries.[26, 27]

Mental health professionals commonly use the term *maladaptive behavior* in describing these same behaviors. Historically, healthcare providers and those who write about IHTs have ignored maladaptive behavior that leads to destructive conflict in IHTs. One of the first articles about maladaptive behaviors on an IHT gave examples of maladaptive behaviors and discussed them as an intrateam phenomenon in terms of willing and unwilling participants as conduits, receptors, and reflectors.[28] The article also gave suggestions on how team members could recognize maladaptive behaviors and address them at the individual, dyadic, and team levels. Prior to publication, this article was rejected several times because reviewers refused to believe that maladaptive behavior was a problem on IHTs. However, upon publication numerous comments from readers indicated that these behaviors were very common indeed.

Maladaptive behaviors exist on a continuum from occasional to common and mild to severe, and they generally become more common and more severe when the person exhibiting them feels stressed.[29] These behaviors do not occur just between nurses and physicians. They can be exhibited by professionals from any discipline toward professionals from the same discipline or to any other discipline. And while there have been calls for more monitoring and regulation, the most effective solution might be more well-developed IHTs where team members stand up for one another and come forward when they observe inappropriate behavior. While more recent articles have addressed overt examples of maladaptive behavior in medical settings, maladaptive behavior is not always overt and is often difficult to capture. Frequently the most covert behaviors, like ignoring a professional's suggestions or even their presence, can be much more stressful than overt remarks witnessed by others.

As social human beings, we all engage in behaviors that can be construed by others as manipulative and potentially maladaptive. Because we value certain power currencies, we formulate our communications in a way to draw people to our viewpoint. When we are stressed, we are more likely to use coercive methods. If those with whom we communicate do not share our values or *perceive* that we don't share theirs, they might view our communication as manipulative. For example, if a team social worker continually refers to his or her job as advocating for patients, the other team members might think the social worker views them as not advocating for patients. This is why it is so important for team members to make their values explicit and teach each other what knowledge they bring to the team. Clarifying positions and perceptions will identify common value systems and help stem some of the maladaptive behavior that will inevitably strike the team.

Behavior that is disruptive or maladaptive and potentially destructive to the team is part of every developing team's fabric. Maladaptive behavior that is sporadic or occurs in a one-time angry outburst can usually be addressed by a one-on-one conversation with the team member who is the source of the behavior and the recipient(s) of such behavior. However, maladaptive behaviors that are surreptitious, frequent, focused on turning one team member against another, or extremely hurtful can cause destructive conflict that will rapidly grow, return a team to a *forming* phase and cause competent team members to exit the team.

Team Members: Active or Passive Participants?

Team members, knowingly and unknowingly, can become active and passive participants in a team's system of maladaptive behavior. If a team member chooses to engage in maladaptive behavior, he or she as *originator* can initiate a message that is sent to a *receptor(s)*. Receptors accept the *originator's* message without question, because the message is consistent with what they believe or because the individual giving the messages exhibits qualities prized by the receptors. *Conduits* transfer messages to other team member *receptors* that may or may not be the intended target of the message. *Reflectors* reflect praise to the *originator*, as a reminder that he or she is valued. All of these keep the maladaptive system going.[30, 31]

Although maladaptive behavior might be associated with certain team members more than others, it can also be heavily influenced by the situation in which the team exists (e.g., non-team-related stress levels of members, the history of the team, the knowledge of supervisors regarding maladaptive behaviors, the stability of the organization, and the support and involvement of the broader organization in the well-being of the team). It is sometimes necessary to look at the use of power currencies and maladaptive behavior at a system level, where outside forces might be undermining the fundamental purpose of the team.

BOX 7.9   A WEB OF MALADAPTIVE BEHAVIOR

A nursing assistant (NA) who valued efficiency finished her patient care duties before all of the other nursing assistants. A supervisor complimented the nursing assistant for being so efficient and recommended her to the administrator for a special award. Another NA resented the attention given to the efficient assistant. The slower assistant as the *originator* appealed to the caring nature of several other assistants and, using them as *receptors* and *conduits,* mentioned that she felt the assistant who had received the award did not spend enough time with patients and really did not care for them. These words changed the viewpoints of other NAs, who passed along these negative comments and actively excluded the efficient NA from their breaks, lunches, and parties. They also agreed to collectively work at a slower pace. As this collective behavior intensified, some of the other nursing staff wanted to complain but were convinced by the slower NAs that the efficient NA didn't take enough time with patients and didn't really care about them. Since the NAs seemed united, the nurses believed them. The nurses and other team members chose not to talk with the efficient NA because they didn't want to offend the other NAs. The efficient NA became very distraught and decided to take a job in the kitchen.

Using Conflict to Develop and Maintain the Team

Distinguishing between Relational, Task, and Process Conflict

Sorting through conflict and determining what is destructive from what is potentially creative can be a difficult endeavor. Any conflict can be destructive to the team's work if it is prolonged and unaddressed. However, relational conflict can become particularly troublesome to IHTs if it is not recognized early in its inception. The most important step in acknowledging relational team conflict is to recognize certain behaviors as maladaptive.

Exhibiting arrogance, aggressiveness when criticized, seductiveness, drama, attention-seeking behaviors, excessive charm, coldheartedness, irresponsibility, impulsivity, rage, irritability, self-destructiveness, deceit, or pitting one team member against another are all potentially maladaptive behaviors that can be destructive to IHTs. Identifying these behaviors in teammates is difficult because we usually associate them with certain disorders in patients. However, healthcare professionals can and do exhibit these behaviors. The first step is to recognize and acknowledge the behaviors are occurring. The second step is to determine if and when such behaviors become intense and/or common. Team members must take responsibility to determine if any of these behaviors are negatively affecting the work of the team. If they are disruptive, the team must acknowledge that fact and put established procedures in place to address the team member and initiate efforts to correct the behavior. If efforts fail and the behavior continues the team member should be dismissed. This process must be an ongoing and accepted part of maintaining the team.

It is not safe to assume that the formal leaders of an IHT will be the ones to recognize and address team conflict, because to do so might be perceived by them as failure. Conflict is usually first recognized by those team members who are closest to it or most deeply affected by it. The members who are affected first might also be those who have assumed few informal leadership tasks, because they are the ones who are most intensely watching and learning. The leadership tasks of judge, process analyzer, facilitator, challenger, and reviewer are most helpful for recognizing and addressing relational conflict. However, because these tasks are some of the most difficult leadership tasks, there might be IHTs that have no members willing or able to consistently assume them. If these tasks are left unfilled, there is a high probability that a team will, at some point, become embroiled in unproductive relational conflict, and that conflict could end up destroying the team.

Administrators can be very helpful when they assume leadership for conflict management, particularly relational conflict. However, because so much team conflict is covert, administrators usually do not get involved until conflicts have escalated. Therefore, some team members must be identified and trained to assume these leadership tasks. Any team member should feel safe in revealing their negative experiences to these designated team members.

Task and process conflicts can be important sources of innovation for team decision making.[32] These conflicts can either force team members to search for better solutions to underlying problems, or they can lead to mediocre or undesirable solutions. Producing innovative solutions depends on encouraging and capturing creative suggestions early in their development, even if they provoke conflict. Establishing safe venues for expressing task and process conflicts is one of the most useful things that a team can do. However, establishing them can be tedious.

In a study of a developed IHT, a feeling of comfort with the team was one of many variables associated with assuming and teaching team leadership tasks.[33] Promoting healthy disagreement in the form of constructive confrontation is a leadership task for advanced team leaders. And yet, if members do not feel safe, they will never assume these difficult tasks. It is a major challenge for an IHT to establish the team with structure and process mechanisms in place for acknowledging conflict.

The team can teach all new members how to recognize and address conflict and how to engage in one-on-one constructive confrontation at the interpersonal level. New team members with skills in handling conflict can be targeted to learn and quickly assume specific leadership tasks that identify conflict at the intrateam and interteam levels. Meetings can be designed to allow time to address conflicts, particularly those related to task or process conflict. Rules can be established that do not discourage conflict or the acknowledgment of it. Members can be trained to look for team metaphors or slogans that either encourage or discourage conflict, and to make use of those that encourage constructive confrontation. For example, the slogan "United we stand, divided we fall" might increase cohesiveness but will not likely enhance creative efforts. "United we stand, challenged we succeed" might send a more effective message.

Monitoring and Managing Team Conflict

It is helpful for team members to stand back and analyze conflict situations. By doing this, members may discover they are using an approach that no longer fits the situation or maybe never did. Values, procedures, or structures can keep a team from an impasse when there is too much or too little conflict. Table 7.3 is a guide that will help team members know what interventions are needed in many types of conflict situations.

One strategy in maintaining a team is to assign a team facilitator to monitor and manage conflict. It is often most effective to choose someone as facilitator who is not a clinical member of the team. Unfortunately, not being a practicing clinician on the team excludes the facilitator from the most valued status of *member*. While this makes it more difficult for the facilitator to gain legitimacy with the team, such individuals will quickly prove their worth because conflict is just around the corner. If the facilitator is a team member, that individual must be given time to perform that role. This is a difficult role, and it takes time to monitor a team and provide counsel to its members. If this role is added on to an already

Table 7.3 **Promoting Constructive Conflict on Interprofessional Health Care Teams**

Team Domains	General Approaches	Approach for Too Much Conflict	Approach for Too Little Conflict
Values	Clarify differences and similarities between professional and team values.	Focus on interdependence of team members.	Emphasize importance of open questioning in a learning environment.
	Establish team culture of teaching and learning.	Review dynamics and costs of escalation.	Clarify dynamics and costs of avoiding.
	Increase awareness of feelings and perceptions.	Share perceptions and clarify issues as a team.	Raise consciousness about informal leadership.
Process	Modify within-team procedures.	Increase expression of within-team cohesion.	Increase expression of within-team differences.
	Train team leaders to monitor team climate.	Expand collaborative strategies.	Teach constructive confrontation.
	Monitor team behavior.	Teach members skills of process analyzer.	Teach members the skills of process analyzer.
Structure	Encourage organizational interventions.	Use organizational hierarchy.	Exert pressure for better performance or new approach.
	Develop rules for team membership.	Establish rules for interactions.	Eliminate procedures that stifle conflict.
	Create new roles for team communication.	Integrate overlapping roles of disciplines.	Assign leadership tasks of challenger, judge, process analyzer.
	Redefine team boundaries and goals.	Redesign team to emphasize task.	Clarify tasks for informal leadership in patient care and team process.

overburdened practitioner, it will quickly fall to the wayside. Ideally, the facilitator would be someone who is trained in interpersonal dynamics and who understands the nature of IHTs. Such people are difficult to find, and they may be seen as expendable when budgets are cut. If health-care organizations are serious about the value they place on teamwork, they should think not only about establishing IHTs, but also about the costs, benefits, and efficiencies of maintaining teams once they have been established.

BOX 7.10   RULES FOR HEALTHCARE TEAMS

1. Commit to establishing a climate of questioning and open discussion.
2. Everyone has an obligation to disagree if they feel they can improve on an intervention.
3. Everyone has the obligation to give each other honest feedback, for example, "my perception of your role on the team is . . .; I appreciate it when you . . .; It bothers me when you . . ."
4. Disagree at the cognitive level (e.g., focus on tasks and on differences about how to best achieve common objectives) vs. the affective level (e.g., focus on personal incompatibilities or disputes).
5. Recognize that there may be several valid approaches to a situation.
6. Each member teaches new members the mission, values, and norms of the team.
7. Team members follow through on commitments made at meetings.
8. The team establishes a plan to evaluate itself on an ongoing basis.
9. Start and end meetings on time; minimize distractions (e.g., silence electronic devices or only use them in ways that relate to the meeting).
10. Use meetings for issues that need to be discussed by the full team; presentations to the team are direct and to the point.
11. Separate patient care meetings from administrative team meetings.
12. Use agendas and assign someone the responsibility for each item before the meeting.
13. One person talks at a time, while the others listen and don't interrupt.
14. Create solutions that benefit as many parties as possible.
15. Assign complex issues to subgroups to bring new information back to the team.
16. Draft agenda for the next meeting at the end of each meeting.
17. Establish action plans for unresolved problems.

18. On areas of conflict, continue open discussion outside the meeting only among team members involved in the conflict and those with interest in resolving it.
19. Review and evaluate each meeting, for example, have each member say several words about what went well and what could be improved, or unfinished business.

Establishing Team Standards/Values for Conflict

Creating rules for conflict management is extremely important and can be done early in a team's formation. A team will want to re-evaluate these rules as it matures. Teams often ignore establishing standards for conflict management by using some of the avoidance strategies already mentioned. Because conflict management is not a priority when all seems calm, the establishment of standards might not get done at all. A team might not see the value of having standards for conflict management until a major conflict paralyzes the team. Box 7.10 is a set of rules that could provide a team with ideas on what they might want in their practice standards. These rules are only suggestions. It is most useful if each team establishes its own rules and the members agree to adhere to them. The standards should be clarified for prospective team members before they agree to join the team.

Summary

Healthcare professionals are well trained but they are not robots. They can be hurt by disruptive and maladaptive behaviors, and they need time and opportunity to resolve their conflicts. Conflicts can be constructive or destructive, and often the most destructive conflicts are caused by behaviors that are either covert or conflicts that are ignored by other members of the team. Managing conflict on IHTs involves changing professional culture and human behavior. Identifying and resolving team conflicts should be established as part of the culture of an IHT. Healthcare professionals need permission, time, and opportunity to resolve team conflicts when necessary.

If a team's culture develops based on principles of individual professional culture and autonomy, the team is not interprofessional and will probably not see any value in interprofessional conflict. Although a team's culture is not a tangible commodity, it will be understood by the team's members and is one of the first things that a new member will notice. Establishing rules for team conflict is helpful, but it is not sufficient to assure that a team will use conflict to its advantage. An IHT that is well functioning will, over time, develop a culture that values conflict. In fact, the value a team has for conflict will become part of that team's culture. An IHT that is well functioning will have a culture that views conflict as an essential element for team growth and innovative problem solving.

Questions for Discussion

1. What are some conflicts your team has experienced?
2. How does your team usually address conflicts?
3. What kinds of conflicts do different members of your team feel comfortable addressing?
4. If you observed your team pharmacist ignoring the advice of one of the team nurses, what would you do?

8

The Patient as Teacher and Learner

The nature of a patient's relationship to the IHT always has an element of uncertainty. Patients differ in their levels of education, knowledge of health care, values related to healthcare practices, and past experiences with healthcare professionals and systems. Although patients benefit from being involved in their care,[1] the level of involvement patients desire will differ. The presence or absence of mental health issues like dementia, anxiety, or paranoia will also affect the patient's relationship with the IHT. Factors like severe pain and receiving a new diagnosis or diagnosis of a serious disorder can distort even a well-informed patient's ability to absorb information. An enhanced level of assistance in helping patients understand their condition can improve outcomes and reduce costs.[2] In addition to assessing a patient's general level of healthcare knowledge, it is important for team members to remain vigilant to a patient's ability to hear and understand what is being said. It is common for healthcare professionals to either underestimate or overestimate a patient's ability to process information about their health problems. It is the responsibility of the IHT to ascertain a patient's mental capacity, level of understanding, and how much involvement a patient desires for healthcare decision making.

Just as patients differ in their knowledge of health care and teamwork, healthcare professionals differ in their knowledge of teams and the benefits of a team approach for patients. Also, well-developed and highly functional IHTs exist within systems of healthcare delivery that may or may not be amenable to patients' involvement in their health care. According to the World Health Organization 1948 Universal Declaration of Human Rights, there are at least four models of health care that depict the patient–physician relationship in the United States and Europe, that is, *paternalistic, informative, deliberative,* and *interpretive.*[3]

Ethicists debate about which models are appropriate in varying situations. Patients, healthcare professionals, administrators, politicians, and insurers operate according to these models, and each model has value in health care. Some entities promote the models in their pure form, and others combine models depending on their needs. It is doubtful that patients, healthcare professionals, or healthcare systems discuss or even realize their model preferences, but those preferences profoundly affect the way health care is sought by patients and delivered by healthcare professionals. Table 8.1 describes and extrapolates these four models as they might relate to patients and IHTs in the current U.S. healthcare environment.

Table 8.1   **Models of Health Care as They Relate to the Patient/IHT**

Model	Description	Views Patient As	Expectations of Patient	Expectations for IHT
Paternalistic	MD/NP/PA judges what is best for patient	Child or incapable	Low	Low
Informative	Patient is responsible for obtaining medical information and makes all decisions	Consumer	High	Uncertain
Deliberative	Outcomes research creates framework for treatment	Subject	Low	High
Interpretive	Interpersonal processes between patient and IHT prescribe and support care	Participant/ partner	Moderate	High

Source: Extrapolated from World Health Organization models of patient–physician relationship (http://www.who.int/genomics/public/patientrights/en/).

Models of Healthcare and Teamwork

Paternalistic Model

In the *paternalistic* model of health care, the health professional is expected to do what is best for the patient, and sometimes the perceived needs of the patient are usurped by the needs of society. *Paternalism* can become problematic when a healthcare provider who does not have all the information needed to solve a patient's problems makes definitive decisions about that patient's care. Patients have become the focus of marketing efforts by healthcare providers, pharmaceutical companies, and insurers. The ads are intended to convince patients they have the power to choose their own medicine or are equal partners with their healthcare team. The phrases, *talk to your doctor* (about whatever product is being advertised); *patient–physician partnership*; *patient-centered care*; and *patient-as-team-member* are commonly used and make it appear as though patients are in control. However, there is little agreement on the meaning of these phrases, and patients see plenty of evidence that they are not in control of their health care. While these slogans make for great sound bites, much of health care still operates in a paternalistic environment.

Websites for healthcare systems use terms that describe patients' rights. These terms include the words *respect, quality, clean, safe, privacy protection, help with claims*, and *patient involvement*. The Agency for Healthcare Research and Quality (AHRQ) has a special section on its website for patients and consumers. The section begins with the following statement: "Get more involved with your health care by asking questions, talking to your clinician, and understanding your condition. Patients and families who engage with healthcare providers ask good questions and help reduce the risk of errors and hospital admissions."[4] Unfortunately, even when patients try to get more involved in their health care by attempting to assert a place within the team, their attempts might be rejected, as the following case illustrates.

> **Joan:** "I called for a yearly physical. I was told to come in a week ahead of my wellness visit for blood work despite me telling them I had already had the blood work done for free at my job. In the past I had been told to write down all of my questions and all my medicines. So when I was asking my questions and concerns I had my list of questions in a folder on my lap. After answering a couple of my questions the doctor asked if he could take my folder from me. I said I think I have covered some things but not all of them. The doctor then said he was told he was no longer supposed to answer questions at these wellness visits. He said they didn't have time for

all this because the team has a lot of things to get through. He said I would have to make another appointment. Everyone I have told this story to has said they had been told the same thing. Plus the doctor was a half hour late already. He yelled at me and I didn't get any of my questions answered. This visit was a waste of my time. And this was an award winning diabetes doctor. In the short amount of time I was there the doctor spent all his time correcting my data in the chart. They are so intent on checking off things they need to do that the patient gets lost in the process."

Joan's example represents a *paternalistic* model of health care and a lost opportunity to help her toward better health. Wellness visits are perfect opportunities for teams to engage patients in their care and to work on agreements for improving or maintaining health. Changes in health care that have occurred over the past 15 years may have increased efficiency at the expense of challenging the provider–patient relationship. In the past, the physician most commonly judged what was best for the patient, prescribed a procedure or method of care, and made sure the patient received that care.

The *paternalistic* model of health care remains strong. However, control has shifted from the healthcare professional to the institutions that employ health professionals and also to the health insurance providers. This institutional *paternalism* is making patients question who is responsible for their care. Ever-changing controls on what diagnostics or medications patients are allowed cause patients to lose trust in healthcare professionals and the teams in which they work. This emerging *paternalism* also leaves patients and members of IHTs questioning their roles in the process of healthcare delivery.

Informative Model

In the *informative* model, the patient is viewed as a consumer of health care. Theoretically, patients receive comprehensive medical information and are expected to make all decisions related to their health care. Under the extreme manifestation of this model, patients would receive a certain amount of money for their health care and would be expected to obtain and compare costs of procedures provided by different institutions. Patients would also be expected to compare performance scores among teams of professional providers. This is the model favored by some politicians and economists.

Problems with the *informative* model include an inability to accurately measure performance, since many healthcare outcomes can be subjective.

Currently, a large piece of performance evaluations is patient satisfaction scores. In pursuit of the positive evaluations that will bring institutions more money, some hospitals offer amenities commonly seen in loyalty programs for hotels.[5] Unfortunately, ill patients do not always know what is in their best interests and, blinded by the bling, might give a hospital stay or medical encounter a higher rating than it deserves. Also, hotel or theme park management principles do not necessarily apply to good health care.

Another unfortunate element of the *informative* model is it can be a form of *paternalism* under the guise of informing the patient. It has the potential to woo patients with marketing strategies without their awareness of potential costs to their health care. Also, proponents of this model rarely discuss its psychological costs to healthcare professionals who feel they need to please administrators who might be more focused on the bottom line than on promoting better health care. Incomplete information can become a double-edged sword. As patients learn about new treatments through advertisements and the Internet, it puts pressure on the healthcare system and the system pushes back in the form of increased *paternalism*. Insurance providers repeatedly deny requests from physicians for specific medicines, recommended tests, and requested procedures. This leaves the patient in limbo and weary medical providers in a quandary.

When insurers deny requests, often patients must act as their own advocates, and that is a role most patients are not trained to perform. Insurance boards of 5–10 members only meet periodically, and appearing before them is intimidating for most patients. In many cases, the insurance boards that deny services do not have the required expertise to deny a service, and instead use general interpretations of a procedural manual to make their decisions. In addition, administrative requirements often overwhelm healthcare professionals, so they don't have time to provide the information necessary for a patient's appeal.

Healthcare insurers might only focus on one test or procedure, without accounting for how it relates to a patient's complex health picture that should dictate what the patient really needs. The following letter by Dr. Smith illustrates what it takes to win an appeal before a review board. Despite being told repeatedly by her physician that the insurance review board had never rescinded a decision to deny a patient coverage for a procedure, a retired physician used her knowledge of health care and the help of her providers in appealing the board's refusal to fund a procedure she thought was necessary to proceed with her care.

Dear Healthcare Review Board Members:

I reviewed the letter declining to cover genetic testing for FHH. Thank you for the opportunity to respond. I interpret "Medical Necessity" as being met by a single *positive* criterion, rather than being denied by a single *negative* criterion. In my case criteria "e." is positive. [Individuals with the phenotype of FHH whose parents are/were both normocalcemic—i.e., FHH possibly caused by a de novo CaSR mutation.]

May I assume that you feel that a 24-hour urine collection with a calculated calcium/creatinine of .007 in my case [criteria d.] is diagnostic of FHH with no need for confirmative genetic testing. I believe the .007 value is suggestive of FHH but not diagnostic, especially without a family history. Can you provide me with citations and medical literature indicating that this test is diagnostic without genetic confirmation? I performed a Medline on the diagnosis of FHH. Based on this review I conclude that the calcium/creatinine clearance ratio is a first-step screening test. Diagnosis of FHH requires genetic testing. See below.

[paragraphs deleted]

Therefore, I believe that a 24-hour urine determination for calcium/creatinine should be considered a screening test. Please reconsider the denial of genetic testing for FHH. If the genetic test is diagnostic of FHH, I will not pursue additional parathyroid surgery to correct my systemic abnormality. Currently the diagnosis of FHH is tenuous and uncertain. There is no family history consistent with this diagnosis. My physicians and I will be forced to consider additional imaging and minimally invasive surgery to prevent the adverse effects of possible diffuse hyperparathyroidism. Thanks for your consideration. Along with my endocrinologist, I plan to attend the appeals hearing via Skype.

Sincerely,

Rene Smith

Several days after this letter was sent to the appeals board, the procedure was approved and the hearing was canceled. Rene's case was unusual because, as a retired physician, she had the time and knowledge to garner the information needed to refute the insurance board's decision. It is also unusual because the board overturned its original denial. The fact that Rene's physician was willing to appear before the board indicated a level of teamwork that likely influenced the board's decision. Cases like this occur many times a day in healthcare settings. They also occur at higher levels where claims reviewers for Social Security are paid according to the number of claims they deny. Hospital administrators must hire people whose sole responsibility is to build cases that refute these denials of service. It is easy to see how patients, healthcare providers, and administrators can benefit by working together as a team in ensuring appropriate and effective health care. Challenging activities that don't promote better health care is a teaching role that all parties must assume.

Deliberative Model

In the *deliberative* model, the team, including administration, creates a framework for research-driven approaches to care. The outcomes of the research are used to set standards for professionals and their teams to follow. It is the model many healthcare systems have aspired to in the recent past. Driven by the need for increased safety in health care, the Institute for Healthcare Improvement (http://www.ihi.org) has developed and heavily promoted the deliberative model. In general, sound research should always drive better health care. One of the problems with this model happens when numbers become the solution and those numbers are based on a faulty premise or have collection bias. Public funding for healthcare research has diminished over the past 15 years as more research is being funded by proprietary companies. Also, problems with data quality are common in health care.[6] Data are sometimes interpreted erroneously by clinicians and entered into patients' charts. Newer, up-to-date information is entered, and the old data are not removed. In Rene's situation, the standards being used to judge her case were based on incomplete data. In other situations, individuals who have not been trained in data collection techniques collect data.

There is controversy over the amount of involvement patients should have in their care. Whether or not patients should keep their own charts, see all of the notes in their charts, or not be allowed access to their charts remain gray areas. In a study of 1,406 physicians and other health providers, and 1,102 random Web users who were patients, the patients were 31 percent more likely than physicians to say the patient rather than the physician owned their medical records.[7]

> **Joel:** "When I visit my doctor, the clinic assistant has the responsibility for checking my medications. Occasionally I will be lucky enough to get an assistant who wants to ensure the data in my chart is correct and that individual will review my history. Every time this happens I discover my chart is full of errors, things like the number of my siblings and their ailments to the causes of my parents' deaths. And just when I think the information has been corrected, I will be faced with new misinformation. If it is so difficult to correctly record my biographical data, it must be impossible to accurately record my health data."

Rita: "I had just moved to a new city and had to change to a different healthcare system. The first time I saw my new doctor I brought a copy of all of my healthcare records. They were extensive and I made the mistake of not making a copy for myself. A few weeks later I was referred to a specialty clinic that was not in the same system, and I needed a section of my records. I checked with my new doctor's office to see if they had sent a copy of that section to the specialist. They had not, so I asked them for my records so I could take them to the appointment. I thought they were my property anyway, since I had just brought them in. They said the records were their property and would not let me have them. As I became angrier the volume of my voice increased and I could see I was entertaining the waiting patients. The receptionist finally called the doctor to talk with me, and I left with a copy of my records."

The transition to electronic medical records (EMRs) has not solved the problem of medical record errors. Joel makes a good case for why patients should have access to their charts. They could act as fact checkers to ensure data are accurately recorded. Different healthcare systems use different EMR systems, and, until they are standardized, Rita's case is a reminder that when patients see providers from different systems they are in jeopardy.

Unlike data in other businesses, the data in healthcare are often subjective. Studying outcomes from IHT interventions is no exception. IHTs have an important role to play in health care. However, because of their organic nature, they are difficult to study. It is very difficult to conduct an outcome study on an IHT using a prepost design, because the independent variable, the IHT in a real-life setting, is constantly changing. For example, if an IHT is in the *performing* phase at the beginning of an outcome study, and during the study key team members are transferred to other departments, causing the team to revert to the *norming* phase, the outcomes of the study will likely be affected. Unless the study design accounts for or protects against this possibility, the study results will not be valid.

Interpretive Model

The *interpretive* model refers to interpersonal processes that support the general health care of individuals. This model has always been a core value of physicians who are general practitioners.[8] Additionally, the *interpretive* approach is a core value of nursing and social work. It is a very useful primary model for an interprofessional team approach to care, while supplementing it with the other three models. The *Wisconsin Star Method*[9] is an example of a comprehensive tool to assist in addressing complexity in patients. It promotes an *interpretive* model while providing a handy structure for team intake, evaluation, and care planning. Team members might assemble their own comprehensive assessment instrument as an exercise in team development. Discovering who the patient is and how best to meet an individual patient's intersecting needs is at the heart of such an assessment.

Using a comprehensive assessment instrument at intake, an IHT has the ability to gather background information on a patient that forms the basis for an integrated problem list and unified treatment plan. As part of the assessment a team member can ascertain patients' desires for team involvement in their care and subsequently negotiate each patient's place relative to the team. Once that is accomplished, patient and team can be active partners in maintaining and improving the patient's health. When well-functioning IHTs are confident in their assessment processes they can even support the patient in challenging an insurer's denial of service for a procedure the team deems necessary.

Giving and Receiving Feedback

Another part of the patient–team partnership is giving and receiving feedback. Soliciting patient feedback is not easy. Also, healthcare providers have to actually want patients' feedback and be willing to act on their concerns. Patients are often willing and capable of learning about their condition, how best to interact with the team, how to ask questions when they don't understand, and how to obtain more information when they feel they need it. If patients aren't actual members of their team, they certainly want to participate with the team in decisions related to their care.

In the interest of unbiased feedback, third-party providers send out patient care surveys. However, patients complain of getting surveys in the mail after a clinic visit or after a surgical procedure that have few questions relevant to their concerns. Timing of surveys is difficult. Patients who receive a survey shortly after returning home from a hospitalization or clinic visit when they are still not feeling well may be unable to relate details of a negative or unsafe incident. However, recovered patients readily forget about negative experiences, so waiting too long to send a survey is also problematic. Members of IHTs can solicit real-time feedback from patients by asking them how they are doing, asking how they perceived their procedure, or asking patients to describe three positives and three negatives about their healthcare experience. It should be the norm to ask patients what you could do better. Perhaps this would start dialogue between patient and providers that could do more than surveys to improve care. It would have the added benefit of making the patient feel part of their care team.

What Patients Want

While an accurate diagnosis is at the top of the list, patients' desires to feel respected and to be heard are major concerns. In talking with patients and reading about their healthcare complaints, it is clear they want to be treated like human beings. They want respect both for who they are and for their time. Often practitioners assume that they are the only ones with time constraints, and they don't take into account how difficult it is for the patient to get to an appointment or how busy the patient might be. Patients readily talk about their healthcare experiences to their friends and significant others. You can learn from asking people you know about their healthcare experiences. In talking to patients about what they want most from their healthcare providers, certain themes emerge.

Meaningful Communication

One of the things patients and caregivers want most is healthcare providers who communicate at their level of understanding. This can refer to the meaning of test results and diagnoses, or it can mean being in touch with the patients concerns and addressing those concerns. Patients and their caregivers have usually had more time than providers to think through their healthcare situations. Patients often get stuck on obstacles providers never consider. The following cases magnify this observation and the need to listen to the patient.

Ira: "Why are we so grateful for polite human behavior from healthcare providers? Is it because we don't expect it and are shocked when it occurs?"

Robert: "I am thinking of filing a complaint with the practice manager about this last appointment. It was a waste of time. I had to wait 2 weeks because the MD was on vacation. I emailed on my patient portal asking about the purpose of the appointment, but I received no reply. I then called and asked and was told the doctor wanted to give me my MRI results. I said it is a long way to drive just for that, but was told the MD would not give results over the phone. I had to wait over half an hour in a very small room and never did see the doctor. The doctor's assistant came in and told me my results were negative and they have no idea what is causing my pain. I think they could have emailed or called for that. It was annoying."

If the members of this clinic had been working as an IHT, they would have developed procedures for delivering negative test results in ways that accommodated patient's needs. Also, they would have discussed in advance with the patient the roles of the team's members, which members of the team might contact the patient, and which forms of communication were preferable.

To Be Seen as Adults

Patients want to be seen as adults with lives and time constraints. Patients who have to take off work, hire a babysitter, or request transportation services for a medical appointment rightly believe their time is valuable. Patients don't want to be ignored because they are old, or female, or from a different culture, or just because they are patients. If the rules of engagement don't make sense, patients get upset. Patients want reasonable control over their care.

Anne: "I am 85 years old and live alone in my home. My daughter noticed a large bump that had formed on my elbow and took me to the urgent care center. I felt irritated when the doctor ignored me and directed questions to my daughter. The doctor said she would send the aspirate for analysis since it had blood in it. She gave me a prescription for pain and told me she would call in a week, and I should make an appointment for two weeks. A week went by and the doctor did not call. I kept my two-week appointment and was seen by a different doctor. The doctor said that he knew nothing of the aspiration, as there was no note in the chart nor could he find a report of the test. He listened to my story and told me he would check on the results of the test and I should make an appointment for two weeks. I was sure I had cancer and that neither the doctor nor my daughter wanted to tell me.

I returned in two weeks and a third doctor saw me. That doctor found nothing in the chart about either the aspiration or analysis done 4 weeks prior. He told me he would check to see what the problem was and I should make an appointment for two weeks. I angrily said I would not make an appointment until they found the results of the test. While checking out I told my story to the receptionist, who said she would look into it and call me and at that point they would make an appointment. Within an hour of arriving home the receptionist called and told me on the day of the test the nurse had come into the room and accidentally disposed of the specimen.

I asked for the phone number of the physician who drew the sample to ask why she didn't tell me the test was lost. The physician dismissed me by saying, 'Everyone makes mistakes.' I never returned to the clinic."

Janine: "I don't understand why some healthcare providers are caring and others are not. When I was in the hospital the surgeon sat down, looked me in the eye, and he answered my questions. He made me feel like a person. Also, the way the neurosurgeon treated me in the clinic was phenomenal. He also sat down, looked at me, and he had a sense of humor. I told him I wanted to take my neck brace off. He said he understood and then proceeded to tell me what the consequences would be and let me make the decision."

Patients want to be listened to and have their concerns taken seriously. Patients shouldn't have to be surprised when their healthcare provider sits down, looks them in the eye, and reacts thoughtfully to what they say. Although patients with grade school educations might have different levels of understanding from those with master's degrees, patients generally know what bothers them. And life experience can impart a lot of knowledge. Healthcare providers must not only ask questions about patients' backgrounds, but also those responses must be in a prominent place in the chart so any member of the team can place themselves at the patient's level of understanding. It is the responsibility of an IHT to account for the life experiences of patients when engaging them in their own care.

Team members' obligations to the team should match their obligations to the patient. The receptionist, nursing assistant, nurse, and physician are all part of the team. Someone from the team should have called Anne back to obtain another sample. In speculating on the reasons no one took proper action, one could blame a lack of experience, a lack of trust between team members, or fear on the part of a team member. Whatever the reason for not addressing this mistake, the team did not take responsibility for meeting the needs of this patient. It was the receptionist who finally assumed a leadership role in discovering the source of the problem. The physician was correct in telling Anne that everyone makes mistakes. However, if the team had been functioning well, someone would have reported the mistake and a well-functioning IHT would never have allowed this mistake to mushroom out of control.

The Patient as Teacher

Failure to Listen

If we listen hard enough, we find patients can be great teachers. As I speak with patients, I find one of their biggest concerns is having their healthcare providers not listen to them or ignoring concerns that relate to their health. The case of Ruth Saxon in Chapter 1 (see Box 1.1) reflects this concern. Not only did the team fail to respond to Ruth's apparent uneasiness, they totally ignored George's pleas for help that related back to his being able to keep his wife in the long-term care facility. On the surface this story appears to reflect a lack of compassion and an absence of leadership among the team's members. However, it is more likely that it was a lack of collective knowledge about how to address this couple's complex problems, plus a lack of focus on the team's overarching goal for Ruth.

Health care has evolved with increasingly cumbersome rules and regulations. Healthcare providers who are not highly trained will sometimes focus more on making sure they have met administrative requirements. Their goal becomes checking their required tasks or meeting established quotas, instead of delivering care to the patient. Every team needs leaders who can function as teachers by assuring the team listens to patients. Often a team's best teachers come in the form of seasoned clinicians. These clinicians can help team members understand what the patients are trying to teach them.

> **Leslie:** "I am a nurse on a general medical unit in a hospital and was making patient rounds at about 9 a.m. when an elderly gentleman who had a cancer diagnosis told me he wanted to be a DNR (do not resuscitate). I asked him if he had told his doctor. His response was negative, so I told him I could get it taken care of for him. I asked the patient what he was thinking and if he had a reason to be concerned. He said he just needed to get it done. I went to talk with the patient's physician who didn't want to do it then. By 11:30 a.m. the patient was dead. The doctor came and asked me how I knew. Subsequently that physician came to me and said he learned that he needed to listen to the patient."

> **Oscar:** "Sam was in his early 90s when he was admitted to the hospital for the umpteenth time. Sam was an alcoholic and extremely cachectic. The team had been struggling with how they could creatively get nutritious calories into him, since most of his calories were consumed in the form of alcohol. As the team social worker, I had been working with Sam's daughter to see if we could stop the liquor deliveries to Sam's apartment. I reviewed the chart and realized the Resident on the unit had prescribed two shots of brandy a day for Sam. When I confronted the Resident he said Sam had wheeled himself to the Director's office to complain about his care. Because the Director's father had been Sam's army buddy, the Director listed to Sam's request for two brandies a day. When I spoke to the Resident who wrote the orders, he said he didn't see anything wrong with Sam

having two drinks a day since he was probably going to die soon anyway. I then asked the Resident if he knew what Sam's goal in life was. He gave me a strange look when I suggested he pose the question to Sam. The next day I again spoke to the Resident and he said he had rescinded the order for alcohol because Sam told him his goal was to make it to 100 so his name would be announced on the Today Show. Sam's name was not mentioned at 100 but he died shortly after it was announced on his 102nd birthday."

Listening is one of the most important elements in communicating with a patient. Discovering the essence of what the patient is telling you can be very difficult. Sometimes it is what the patient doesn't say that is most important. Frequently it is another team member who understands the patient's most important needs, and that individual must be strong enough to help the team understand the patient's message.

The Patient as Learner

Encounters with Uncaring Behaviors

Uncaring behavior by healthcare professionals has multiple causes and takes many forms. Extreme stress or fatigue is a major cause. Drug or alcohol abuse can be another cause. Sometimes healthcare providers enter their profession for the wrong reasons and end up taking it out on patients. More commonly, some healthcare providers do not have the knowledge required to compassionately address a patient situation. Team members and administrators must be on guard for clues to potentially hurtful behavior by their colleagues. Whatever the causes of uncaring behaviors, it is the patients who usually suffer the most.

Rita: "I was discharged from the intensive care unit to a rehab unit after suffering a broken neck and multiple fractures. Every evening a nursing assistant (NA) would enter my room and order me to roll over. I was unable to do it by myself, and she just stood and taunted me. One night a different NA came in and asked me to roll over. I told him that I could not, and he gave me several helpful tips that made it easier for me to roll over and sit up. He said he had learned the techniques from a physical therapist with whom he had worked."

Sue: "I am a nurse who had just finished my last shift before a major holiday. My husband, Jim, picked me up from work and we were broadsided on a side street close to home. Jim lost consciousness and I was dazed, but knew that something was very wrong. We were taken to the nearest hospital emergency department (ED) where we were each checked out by different teams. The ambulance crew must have noticed my nametag from work and told the ED team I was a nurse. Someone from the team commented that I would get the same care as anyone else. The team physician came in and was very brusque. I told the physician I had to work the holiday. And he retorted with a question asking me if I was trying to get the holiday off. By this time I was angry and told him he didn't know anything about me, and that his comment was very unfair. He did not know that I had offered to cover for someone else for the holiday. The physician told me he would write an excuse for the holiday but not the day after.

Although I could barely move, the X-Rays were negative. The X-Ray technician was the only staff member who was nice to me. A member of the team came in to discharge me without asking me how much pain I was having. No one said get up and walk so they could observe me. No one said that I had a bruise all the way down my right side. You would think they would say something about it. I didn't get any instruction. I don't deal with car accident patients, so I wasn't sure what I should do. Our daughter was there by then and she had to dress me and help me stand up.

Jim was placed in another exam room. He had a little bruise from a seatbelt over his liver and a very kind nurse. The ED team that took care of Jim did the whole court press on him. Jim got excellent instructions and they wheeled him out on a gurney while I walked alongside him. Both of us were told to make appointments with our primary care providers after the holiday.

After the holiday I called work and told them I couldn't walk, and they told me not to come to work. My primary care physician said my X-Rays were negative, and I just needed PT. I called PT and they gave me an appointment for three weeks from then. I hobbled around for another two weeks and finally called my primary care doctor who got me into PT the next day. The PT was very nice, although when he came in drinking a cup of coffee I asked him to go out and wash his hands and start over. After examining me he said something was really wrong. I was supposed to come back to see him in 2 days but received a call that I would need to see another PT, because the first one had fallen and broken his hand. So I saw another PT, and she repeated that something was really wrong and called in another therapist. They examined me and instructed me to call my primary doctor and tell her I needed a bone scan.

My primary doctor told me she was referring me to Rheumatology, but she would order the bone scan if I insisted. My appointment for the bone scan was on a Monday in two weeks and my appointment in Rheumatology was in 6 weeks. I went for the scan and they injected the dye into my arm and told me to look up and I would see an area on my back that should light up. However it didn't light up. The dye had infiltrated into my arm and they didn't have any more and so I had to wait for more dye to come. When I was finished I checked with the Radiologist who told me to be really careful. On Tuesday I called and left a message that I would like the results of the test. When I didn't hear anything by Wednesday I hit rock bottom and just decided I wasn't going to get better. Then I remembered seeing something in the doctor's office that if things are normal you will get a letter, so I expected a letter.

Thursday, five weeks after the accident, I received a call from my doctor saying I had multiple pelvic fractures and I should stop PT and go to bed. After that they were very attentive and did multiple follow-up scans. I feel if just one of the practitioners I saw had asked me to get up and walk when they saw me they would have known something was terribly wrong. My primary care physician never apologized. I did receive a survey about my ED visit and responded to that. After this resolved I had chest pain during the night and I waited until morning because I dreaded going to the ED but when I finally went in the morning; they were great."

Rita was a patient who was eager to learn how to help herself. She just needed a capable teacher. The case of Sue and Jim is notable because of the contrast in the way they were treated by two different teams in the same ED. The reasons for the uncaring behaviors exhibited by Sue's treatment team are unknown. However, it is evident that the uncaring attitudes had a serious effect on Sue's future behavior when she delayed a trip to the ED for chest pain. Just as you can teach healthcare students how to interact with patients, you can offer tips to patients on how to interact with the healthcare system and the IHT. However, what is learned will come more from observed behavior than from the formal teaching experience. The willingness of patients to speak up about their care will be strongly influenced by what they see in the behaviors of their IHT members. Even when healthcare professionals are uncertain about treatment options, communicating their reasoning to a patient can alleviate stress.

Healthcare professionals are schooled in the reasons patients might act out, and they should be ready for such behaviors. However, patients are not prepared for uncaring behaviors from clinicians. Healthcare professionals are human and at times they do not act with kindness, nor do they follow the principles of good patient care. Timely feedback by caring team members can sometimes avert negative consequences from their bad behaviors. One leadership responsibility of an IHT is to monitor the behavior of its members and give responsive feedback or refer to a supervisor when the aberrant behavior is or potentially could be harmful to the patient. If team members refuse this responsibility the patient might decide to assume it. In such a case the consequences can be more severe.

Carrie: "I was 12 hours out of abdominal surgery that left me with a 13-inch incision. A nurse (LPN) helped me stand up and walk the few steps to a chair. After a short period of time I felt faint and asked the nurse to help me up so I could return to my bed. She refused to help me stand up. After begging the nurse to help me, to no avail, I attempted to stand by myself. Feeling a strong pull on my stitches, I finally forced myself into an upright position. Several months later my incision re-opened and I needed another surgery. I blamed the nurse for coldly refusing to help me."

Carrie (post hospital stay): "When I returned home from the hospital I wrote down a few notes about my hospital experience, and after recovering from my initial surgery I wrote a letter to the hospital administrator about the way the nurse had treated me. Although I didn't want to get the nurse in trouble, I was concerned that she would irreparably harm another patient. After I sent my letter I heard she was removed from the surgery floor."

Healthcare professionals need to watch for lack of compassion in team members. Indifferent behaviors might be temporary due to fatigue or excessive stress. However, if the observed uncaring behaviors are frequent and persistent, team members need to act to protect their patients.

The Team as Case Manager

Patients with complex problems feel more secure when they have one contact person to help them manage their care. Patients generally don't realize they can ask for a case manager to help them through the maze of the healthcare system.

Mara: "When I was seen in the ED they immobilized my shoulder. For two weeks I awaited approval for surgery from the insurance provider. During that time I was unable to sleep in a bed because of the pain, but no one looked at my shoulder. The surgeon had told me I didn't need a pre-op physical. When surgery was finally approved I called the hospital, and they said I needed a pre-op. However, my doctor said they couldn't fit me in for a few more weeks. I begged and they overbooked me so I could get the physical. It was a good thing I had said I wanted a case manager. I was told if I hadn't had a case manager I wouldn't have had the surgery. They wouldn't even have looked at the request for the insurance coverage for three weeks. You have to constantly talk and beg, whatever it is. It is not going to happen if you don't."

Unfortunately, case managers are not always available for the patients who need them. However, well-functioning IHTs understand the advantages of assigning a team member as case manager for a patient with complex problems. The case manager might not necessarily be a nurse or a social worker, but he or she could be any team member with the skills that match the patient's needs.

Clear Rules

In addition to being listened to and respected, patients are looking for clear rules. They want to know what to expect from their clinic, hospital, urgent care, and chronic care teams. Patients also want to know what is expected of them when they encounter these teams. Patients want the same rules to apply whether they are male or female, wealthy or poor, well educated or not. Patients want educational materials that apply to their specific condition. They want to know who to call if they have problems, and they expect the person who answers the phone to give them the right answer.

Patients also want seamless communication within and between clinical settings. Because this is generally a macro issue in regard to teamwork, administrators need to be heavily involved in planning for and making this kind of communication happen. Some of these issues played out with the following patient.

> **David:** "As a healthcare provider I don't expect everything to always go as planned. When I returned home at 3 p.m. from day surgery on my shoulder and realized I had severe pain in my eye. I called the surgery center and was told to go to the ED. When I refused I was referred to the anesthesiologist who had assisted at my surgery. I told him I was sure I had suffered a corneal abrasion during surgery. I said I had some eye drops that had been prescribed by an eye doctor for corneal abrasions but that the prescription was expired. The anesthesiologist agreed that it was likely a corneal abrasion and that they sometimes happened when a patient's eyes were taped during surgery. However, he refused to prescribe the eye drops and said I should go to the ED.
>
> Exhausted and refusing to go to the ED, I called the eye clinic. My eye doctor was out for the day and the only doctor in the clinic kindly agreed to fit me in. After waiting two hours to be seen, the doctor took a picture of my eye. The image showed a lateral abrasion across my eye located where the lid margins met. The doctor agreed the abrasion was likely from taping my eyes during surgery and prescribed replacement drops for the expired ones. I left the clinic to fill my prescription and returned home at 7 p.m.

The next morning the nurse from the surgery center called. I had questions about the large pillow that was part of my shoulder brace and also asked about getting off of the narcotics and returning to my normal pain medications. I was told I had to wear the brace at a certain angle exactly as instructed and could not return to my original pain medications for four weeks. Two days later, pain from my brace was preventing me from sleeping, so I called the Nurse Practitioner from the surgery clinic. The NP said I could remove the piece of the brace that was causing me problems. I saw the NP 5 days later for suture removal and she said I could return to my normal pain medications.

This experience left me pondering from a patient's perspective about mixed communications from a variety of healthcare providers. I realized anew the difficulty of managing some of the more complex and sometimes nebulous problems that occur when communication is required between patient and provider. I realized it is essential to safely meld the highly developed skills of surgeons with the technical procedures that accompany surgery. Multiple times providers asked me to repeat my name and birthdate and to identify the surgical site. I was given prophylactic antibiotics to prevent infection and was asked numerous questions about my allergies. I also heard these same details repeated amongst the surgical team members. However, that detail stopped when my surgery ended.

I was grateful nothing serious had gone wrong during surgery. I did not get an infection or go into anaphylactic shock. Surgical and post-surgical providers were extremely kind. However, I had unnecessary pain following surgery, because of questions that did not get asked before surgery and because the staff members at the surgery center were unable to reliably answer my questions and solve my post-surgical problems. Also, they did not refer my questions to the surgeon or the NP at the surgery clinic. When I told the NP about my eye abrasion she was upset that no one at the surgery center had called her. She agreed to suggest using the problem of eye abrasion for a quality improvement project at the surgery center."

The postsurgical problems experienced by David may seem minor to healthcare providers. However, miscommunication between provider and patient during times of transition can cause unnecessary suffering for patients. Often having a seemingly minor issue thoughtfully solved by a provider who cares can relax a patient, relieve them of pain, and allow them to heal. When a patient receives mixed messages and instructions that are not well thought out, they lose trust in their care providers and may choose to ignore any instructions. Because every provider encounters problems they cannot solve, knowledge of what other providers do best is central to accurate and timely communication and referrals among team members.

Irene: "I was brought to my hospital room after back surgery. During the difficult surgery the surgeon had nicked my spinal cord and wrote an order for me to remain flat on my back for several days. I was on a heavy dose of morphine with a bolus pump, despite telling the anesthesiologist narcotics made me sicker than I needed to be. I was determined to get off of morphine as soon as possible, so I began to ask for oral pain medication. The nurse said I needed to eat before I could take oral medication. I asked how I could get food and was told that I needed to order it myself by calling down to the kitchen. My mouth was extremely dry despite drinking large amounts of water. I called the kitchen. Explaining I had to remain flat on my back while I ate, I asked for suggestions of foods that would be easy to swallow. We agreed on cooked carrots and roasted chicken breast cut into small pieces. A food service worker delivered my tray and placed it on a stand on the other side of the room. I requested she place the stand over my bed as I wasn't allowed to move. Not being able to see the tray, I fumbled for the food with my hands. I easily swallowed several slices of carrots. However when I attempted to swallow a piece of chicken it lodged in my esophagus. Unable to breathe, I remember thinking, 'this isn't how I want to die.' Knowing there would be a delayed response to the call button, I forced myself onto my side while jamming my fist into my diaphragm. The chicken popped out. A few days later as I was walking the halls of the hospital I noticed the walls were plastered with quality improvement goals, indicating which ones the hospital was meeting and which ones they were excelling at. This was a well-run hospital clearly focused on improvement. However, no one had picked up on the fact that I shouldn't have been allowed to have solid food while I was forced to lie on my back. I guess that wasn't one of their quality improvement goals for the month."

Irene's story is another example of a transition from surgery to postsurgical care and the lack of team communication. Unfortunately, this story could have had deadly consequences. The decision to have patients call the kitchen to order their own food was likely propelled by an attempt to give patients more control. However, the surgeon's order should have triggered a series of safeguards. In this case it did not and neither the nurses nor the food service workers assumed leadership to recognize the danger cues. Effective quality improvement encourages healthcare providers to be attuned to every situation they encounter, to consider the consequences of their behaviors including their handoffs, and to assume leadership when they see something that doesn't make sense. Patients do want clear rules. However, those rules need to make sense in the context of good health care. And rules that seem clear to healthcare providers should be met with a healthy dose of skepticism. You know an IHT is functioning well when team members feel free to question rules and the decisions of their fellow team members.

Costs to the Patient of Not Working as a Team

Georgia: "I met my friend, Ellen, at the ED. She had been called back after being discharged from the same ED twice in the previous two weeks, being told they couldn't find anything broken from her fall out of bed which caused her to hit her chin on her nightstand. The anti-inflammatory medications the doctors had prescribed were causing Ellen extreme stomach pain. Because of her pain, Ellen was unable to fix meals and hadn't been eating.

Ellen, a severely kyphotic 93 year old, was ushered into a room and immediately informed by the neurosurgeon that her fall had caused fractures at C_1 and C_2 and a bone was pressing on the ligament that separated it from the spinal cord. The surgeon immediately began discussing surgery with Ellen when she started crying and said she did not want surgery. Ellen screamed when the ED nurse placed a neck brace on her and was still crying as she was admitted. As Ellen was admitted to the hospital I had to leave for home several hours away. Driving home I recalled the position of Ellen's nightstand and realized that she had hit her chin, forcing it up and back as she fell. I called the head nurse on Ellen's floor expressing concern the brace was reproducing the mechanism of injury that Ellen had sustained and that is why it was so painful for her. The nurse agreed and said that she had been charting heavily about that problem.

I asked the nurse to call the neurosurgeon for an order to remove the neck brace until they could find a better fit. The nurse refused, saying the surgeon wouldn't listen to her. She then gave me the surgeon's personal number suggesting that I call him. I called and he asked how I got his number. I said the nurse had given it to me because she didn't think he would listen to her. I quickly explained why I was calling and on hearing my concerns, he rescinded his order for the brace. However, in her infinite wisdom as a retired nurse Ellen had already removed the brace."

When a physician prescribes a treatment, it is the responsibility of the appropriate team member to administer that treatment as prescribed. If I suspect that it is the wrong treatment, my willingness to speak with the prescribing physician about it will be dependent on my comfort level with that person, and the culture within the clinical organization of cross disciplinary discussion (i.e., asking hard questions across disciplinary boundaries). If there is no established mechanism for easily doing this, if there is tension between disciplines, or if the clinicians are pressed to the limit, it will not happen. If it is this difficult for clinicians to question their colleagues, it is easy to imagine the difficulty patients have with questioning healthcare providers. You can perform quality assurance studies until the cows come home to determine whether someone is properly receiving their prescribed treatments, but if they are the wrong treatments you are not getting at the source of the real medical error.

Summary

Discussion about models of health care and their meaning for patients and clinicians will continue. Whatever the approach health care takes, patients want the basics of feeling heard and respected as adults who are involved in their healthcare decisions. Patients' natural relationship to the IHT is that of both teacher and learner. Approaching the patient as both teacher and learner can strengthen the power of the IHT not only within itself, but also within the broader healthcare system. Experienced clinicians can be catalysts in this process. Patients don't always know what constitutes good health care and might need to be taught. Healthcare professionals don't always know how to listen to patients in ways that can improve patient care. The patient and the team must become partners in finding the models of care that work best for each patient. Administrators and healthcare systems are partners in this process. They too need to incorporate the true picture of what patients really want and need and learn to work with clinicians to focus on meaningful interventions to promote the best health care possible.

Questions for Discussion

1. In your experience, how involved do patients want to be in their health care?
2. How would you ask a patient how she would like to be involved with her care?
3. What would you do if you saw a patient being mistreated by another healthcare provider?

9

Values and Ethical Issues in Interprofessional Practice: A New Dimension of Teamwork[*]

Introduction

Ethical issues in health care are constantly changing, as they reflect new developments and trends in how care is delivered. Just as IHTs have emerged as an increasingly important form of practice in addressing issues of the cost, quality, and safety of health care in the United States, so too has the recognition of the implications that collaborative practice has for thinking about ethical issues and dilemmas that emerge when different professionals work together on a team. In a previous era of traditionally more independent practice, each professional was primarily responsible for knowing and following his or her own, individual ethical standards. Separate professional organizations reinforced moral guidelines that were discipline-specific. Now, however, with the advent of more team-work practice, it is obvious that we have entered a new era in how ethical

---

[*] Parts of this chapter are based on two previous publications: Clark, P. G., and Drinka, T. J. K. (2002). Exploring responsibility, accountability, and authority in geriatric team performance. In M. D. Mezey et al. (Eds.), *Ethical patient care: A casebook for geriatric health care teams* (pp. 208–229). Baltimore, MD: Johns Hopkins University Press; and Clark, P. G., Cott, C., and Drinka, T. J. K. (2007). Theory and practice in interprofessional ethics: A framework for understanding ethical issues in health care teams. *Journal of Interprofessional Care, 21*: 591–693.

concerns in health care are defined and the moral discourse about how to address them is framed. These issues involve not only how providers relate to their patients, but also how they interact with each other and with healthcare administrators.

Similarly, as we have already discussed, health care in the United States is increasingly dominated by a market model of service provision, with the "business of health care" more and more driving the direction of service development and utilization. As this model also shapes the relationships between providers and patients and between different providers, traditional ethical concerns have increasingly been trumped by economic and efficiency considerations. A focus on economic values has replaced consideration of traditional normative values, leaving both providers and patients to deal with cost savings and profit making as the preeminent factors that dominate health care. The language of business has increasingly replaced that of caring and become the lingua franca of exchanges involving the provision of health services. Even teamwork has increasingly been justified and promoted within a corporate health services administration and management framework.

At their core, traditional ethical concerns involve questions about what is good and bad or right and wrong, and they draw our attention to questions of moral duty and obligation. They also include an examination of the values and principles that guide an individual or a group. In health care generally, ethical issues are usually conceptualized as standards of practice linked to the relationships and responsibilities of individual providers with their patients and other professionals. For example, ethical codes for all major healthcare professions in the United States (such as medicine, nursing, and social work) address these factors. In fact, some codes (such as those for nursing and social work) explicitly call for the responsibility of these professionals to work collaboratively with others in the interest of improved patient care. An important point here is that most ethical issues arise from our relationships with others, whether our patients or our colleagues. It is these relationships that provide the context for ethical concerns to arise and be addressed.

Despite the recognition by some professional bodies of the moral responsibilities of healthcare professionals to act collaboratively, there has been little discussion until recently of the unique ethical competencies required when they work together interprofessionally. Two different organizations, the Institute of Medicine[1] and the Interprofessional Education Collaborative,[2] have developed similar sets of ethical competencies for effective teamwork practice. Healthcare professionals need to have an understanding of both their own and others' values and how these values interact with those of the patient and other professionals. In our experience, such reflection on values, and especially value differences, is seldom practiced and promoted in interprofessional teamwork. Similarly, framing the rights, relationships, and responsibilities among IHT members as ethical issues is rare.

The purpose of this chapter is to explore these emerging ethical issues in interprofessional teamwork, and to develop a simple framework for conceptualizing and organizing them as a start toward recognizing and addressing them when they occur. Doing so requires that we begin this discussion by examining an actual case study illustrating the interface between provider and patient, and focusing on the need for recognizing the importance of values and value differences between professionals. This examination leads to a broader focus on quality of life concerns as they are experienced by different healthcare professionals, including factual and value-laden dimensions.

Then, we will move on to study the critical role that ethics plays within the relationships on the IHT itself and develop a framework that organizes their different levels and dimensions. Taken together, these topics suggest both the centrality of ethics at multiple levels in all of teamwork practice and what the general outline of a new interprofessional ethics might look like and how it differs from the older, single-profession set of ethical guidelines. It is the goal of this chapter to open up a new way of thinking about the requirements of interprofessional practice as having a foundation in moral responsibility.

Defining the Patient's Problem: Clinical Assessment and Values

Setting the stage for this discussion is best done by presenting the initial segment of a case study that illustrates the ethical issues involved in performing an assessment and determining whether a patient has a problem that needs to be addressed by the IHT. We will progressively disclose more of the case as we move through the discussion of ethical issues in IHTs.

Case Study, Take 1: Mr. Robert Crane

You work as a nurse member of an IHT doing geriatric assessment and care plan development within the outpatient clinic of the Geriatrics Department of Shady Grove Hospital in North Southwick. A resident of the community, Mr. Robert Crane, has been scheduled for an initial clinic visit by his daughter, who is concerned about his health and living situation. Other core members of the team include a physician and a social worker; a pharmacist, nutritionist, and physical therapist are "on call" to join the team if their expertise is required.

You perform the initial intake consultation to discuss Mr. Crane's situation with him and his daughter, Mrs. Domenico, who says:

> "I'm really concerned about my Dad—he's 87 years old, you know. He lives alone in his house on Maple Avenue; my Mom died five years ago. He seems to have become more withdrawn during the past year, and seldom gets out anymore. He still does a bit of shopping on his own, but he relies on his neighbors and me more and more for getting groceries and running errands. Dad has been having a lot of trouble recently with getting up and down his outside steps. I don't think that he's eating well either; I look in his refrigerator whenever I visit him, and it looks like all the food we buy him is still in there.
>
> I don't think he talks to anyone from week to week, except his neighbors and me. I think he's lost interest in life since Mom died. He gets a lot of junk mail delivered to the house, and it's piling up in boxes in his living room. He says that he needs to have more time to read it and sort it out. Frankly, I think Dad is 'losing it,' and I'm concerned about his mental state. The house is a mess, with piles of mail everywhere, so that I have to be careful of falling over boxes of it when I walk from one room to the next. The place also smells of cat urine all the time—Dad has six cats!
>
> Dad doesn't think that he has a problem, but I do and I need your help in getting to the bottom of it!"

Facts and Values in Defining a Problem

This case illustrates some fundamental aspects of the values at stake in assessing whether a clinical problem exists and, if so, what are its major components. Different health professionals have differing ways of seeing it and framing its dimensions. Thus, it becomes important for the members of an IHT to become aware of these differences and how they affect the interaction and communication among the different professions on the team.

Every definition of a clinical problem faced by a healthcare professional consists of a factual and a value component. There is no purely "objective" basis for defining a problem in the absence of some value that is potentially affected by the factual state of affairs. For example, we cannot say that the facts of Mr. Crane's living situation are a problem in the absence of some value(s) that might be threatened by his lifestyle. Moreover, value orientations can affect our view of reality and the selection of information that we consider important to defining a problem in the first place.

For example, professionals differ in their logic of clinical assessment—that is, how to gather information from the patient to define the problem. This difference may be thought of as two different styles of practice, one emphasizing "ruling out problems" and the other "ruling in problems." In the former instance, the provider systematically eliminates possibilities until only one problem and a corresponding solution are discovered. In contrast, the latter approach relies on expanding the scope of professional interest to encompass an increasingly long list of potentially relevant factors.[3]

For example, physicians—with their typically more reductionistic values—are trained in diagnostic techniques that narrow down the range of options, relying heavily on "objective" data such as laboratory tests in the process of differential diagnosis. In Mr. Crane's case, for example, the physician on the IHT might order a series of laboratory tests to assess his physical health status. The results of these tests might eliminate certain conditions from consideration, while others might suggest a diagnosis or require further testing. However, in this process "objective" or scientific tests would be the standard for proving or disproving a condition.

Social workers, on the other hand, will focus on Mr. Crane's larger, contextual psychosocial issues, such as income, family relationships, and living arrangements. In this process, they tend to rely on "subjective" data collected by interviews whose interpretations are heavily influenced by clinical judgment and experience. With Mr. Crane, they will want to delve more deeply into his relationship with his daughter, his living arrangement at home, and his own personal wishes to remain autonomous and live the way he wants.

Nurses, depending on their background and training, may fall somewhere between these two extremes. Nurse practitioners tend to be more closely aligned with the biomedical model, whereas clinical nurse specialists have traditionally been considered more holistic in their approach to the patient. Standing between the more "objective" world of medicine and the more "subjective" world of social work, nurses are often described as being more "all encompassing" in their taking into consideration a wide range of the bio-psycho-social aspects of health.

Analyzing these value differences more closely, it is apparent that the traditional orientation of medicine toward the patient may drown out his or her perspective in the process of making clinical assessments, virtually constructing the reality of the patient's condition through powerful medical imperatives to select only the "most important" information; to distance the practitioner from the patient; and otherwise to dehumanize, depersonalize, and decontextualize the patient in the interest of "objective" clinical judgment. Nursing in general and social work, on the other hand, have countervailing pressures to gain a real understanding of the "patient as person," to participate in the patient's world as a way of both understanding it and revealing their own humanity and, even, vulnerability. The approaches of nursing—excluding the more biomedical models of nursing—and social work are more inclusive and holistic than that of medicine.

This difference may lead to a communication gap between professionals, due to the differing assumptions about the importance of incorporating the patient's definition of the "problem" into the clinical assessment process—a theme explored in more depth in Chapter 4. The communication problem here is that a major conceptual gap may exist between professionals and laypersons with regard to their construction of the meaning of health and health-related problems. Providers and patients approach health issues from different perspectives—with the former reflecting the professional and organizational concepts and patterns of clinical practice in which they have been trained, and the latter embodying different influences from their personal experiences, familial contexts, and cultural backgrounds. Though they may use the same words, providers and patients speak different languages.

Moreover, because of differentials in power between the professional and the patient, the professional's definition of need, or the "problem" to be "solved," usually takes precedence over that of the client. The person who controls the definition of the problem simultaneously defines the range of options available to solve it. In other words, recipients of clinical care must have genuine input into the basic construction of need and the concepts used to describe it, or else patients will be prevented from effective dialogue and discussion regarding the important outcomes of the needs assessment process. This is an important feature of patient involvement in interprofessional teamwork.

Insofar as different healthcare professions are trained to emphasize or deemphasize the need for this patient input—depending on their values related to patient autonomy and control over the clinical decision-making process—these differences can be extremely important in distinguishing divergent styles of practice and, consequently, communication problems on IHTs. Nowhere are these issues more apparent than in consideration of quality-of-life issues.

Quality of Life: Using the Same Words But with Different Meanings

Questions of values and value conflicts arise frequently in concerns involving quality of life. By their very nature, considerations of quality of life are at their root value laden and highly individualistic. One person's definition of a poor quality of life may afford another with opportunities to have a very meaningful existence. As people's lives change, their definition of quality of life may shift to accommodate those changes.

Case Study, Take 2: Mr. Robert Crane

Let's follow our initial presentation of the case of Mr. Robert Crane with a second "installment."

In his initial assessment interview, Mr. Crane responds:

"I don't know why I'm here. My daughter dragged me to this meeting! I'm fine! Yes, I live alone, but I'm doing just fine! My daughter helps me with some of the shopping, and I've got some great neighbors who also run errands for me.

I've never been a 'social butterfly' and don't plan on changing now. If I don't see people from one day to the next, that's okay with me. Besides, I have a lot of work to do keeping up with the mail— I get a lot of mail. So, I go through it, each piece—that takes a lot of time! I do feel that my energy level isn't what it used to be, but my doctor has told me that I should expect that since I'm so old.

I don't want to be here for this interview, and I would like to tell you all to get the hell out of my life!"

Communicating around Values in Quality of Life

As Mr. Crane's responses suggest, concerns about quality of life may be in the eye of the beholder, with differences between provider and patient, and, as we will see, between different professionals on the IHT. In assessing these clinically significant differences, it is important that we carefully examine our thought and language and ask the question: "Do we understand and communicate what we really mean?" In particular, personal, professional, and cultural values play an important role in defining and operationalizing the concept of quality of life.

For example, a poor quality of life for one person may be a rich life for another: What we might consider to be a life full of sickness, frailty, and dependence might provide another person with new insights into the existential nature of human life and its continual conditionality and precariousness.[4] Importantly, overemphasis on individual independence in constructing a definition of quality of life may neglect the values of community, collectivism, and cooperation that are equally important in human existence.

Professionals, in particular, differ with regard to their definitions of quality of life—differences with important implications for their ability to communicate over issues affecting clinical decision making. For example, research in long-term care facilities has found that physicians and nursing assistants (whom we may consider to be aligned generally with nursing professional practice models) differ considerably on their feelings about the basis for life-extending treatment and the meaning of care.[5] To the nursing assistants, caring is a more important factor in quality of life than the mental and physical status of the patient; on the other hand, the treatability of a condition tends to be equated by the physicians with higher quality of life for the patient. Differing interpretations of the concept of quality of life underlie these differences in approaches to care. For most physicians, quality of life is related to mental status or freedom from mental impairment; by contrast, quality of life for nurses is more relative. Physical strength, even in the presence of mental impairment, is considered a key determinant of life quality. By contrast, social workers consider the ability of a patient to live where they want to be a major factor in quality of life.

These differences in defining quality of life may be understood within the larger framework of disparities in the perceptions of ethical problems by physicians and nurses. Divergence between these two professions with regard to the recognition of moral dilemmas in practice suggests that such differences are crucial to understanding why communication about value-laden concepts can be so difficult. For example, although physicians and nurses have been found to differ significantly within each of their respective professional groups with regard to how often they perceive ethical dilemmas, nurses more often report conflicts with physicians over ethical dilemmas than do physicians recognize disagreements with nurses.[6]

Other research has also found significant differences between nurses and physicians with regard to the ethical problems they identify.[7] For example, three-quarters of the problems centering on a patient's quality of life were described by physicians rather than nurses. This disagreement over ethical problems is seen as a function of professional orientation and socialization, with nurses increasingly oriented toward patient-centered issues—such as patient preferences, family context, pain control, implementing treatments, and discharge planning. By contrast, physicians are directed more toward problems embodying increased concern about the cost of care and the proper use of medical resources—such as quality of life, economic factors, and inappropriate admissions. Importantly, these physicians' concerns about quality of life are consistent with previous research linking life quality considerations to decisions to withhold therapy, and to the tendency of physicians to rate the life quality of chronically ill elderly more negatively than do their patients.

In addition to medicine and nursing, social work offers us another perspective on the value differences underlying the health professions regarding life quality interpretations. As explored earlier, social work has traditionally represented the broader psychosocial perspective on quality of life concerns in health and illness. This view entails the involvement of several relevant dimensions, including: (1) an assessment of the social environment (including family, social support, economic and cultural factors, and the physical setting); (2) the right of the individual to make his or her own decisions (autonomy); (3) the identification and mobilization of resources in the family and the community; and (4) mediation among the major professional and institutional "players" in defining and solving the individual's "problem."[8] This philosophical orientation ensures that the perspective of the individual on quality of life will be incorporated into the ongoing clinical discussion among the patient, the social worker, and the other health professionals on the IHT.

To summarize, this discussion has highlighted the central importance of personal and professional values in communication between provider and patient, as well as between professionals. Values provide lenses through which we see the world of the patient, critically affect the choice of relevant information about the patient and his or her problem, and set up different discourses about the patient as providers collaborate on the IHT. It is in this latter context that we now consider the emerging level of teamwork ethics.

Developing a Conceptual Framework for Teamwork Ethics

Beyond the level of personal and professional ethics, unique moral issues are beginning to emerge from the growing emphasis on interprofessional education and practice in health care. In order to more fully understand and appreciate the complexity of these ethical concerns, we need first to develop a conceptual framework that provides a structure for their further exploration. It involves the following three elements: (1) *principles* that suggest general behavioral guidelines, (2) *structures* (both formal and informal) that encompass established organizational roles and settings for teamwork practice, and (3) *processes* that are the procedural aspects of ethical practice, focusing on "how things are done" in the healthcare setting. Furthermore, these ethical dimensions can be analyzed at the level of the individual, the team, and the organization. The overall structure incorporating all these factors is displayed in Table 9.1.

Table 9.1　Factors and Levels in an Interprofessional Ethics Framework

Factors/Levels	Principles General guidelines for behavior.	Structures Established forms of knowledge and patterns of behavior.	Processes Procedural aspects of "how things are done."
Individual	• Develop self- and disciplinary knowledge as basis for mutual respect among team members. • Understand norms and practice standards of other professions on team. • Master basic knowledge and skills required for effective teamwork.	• Develop standards of professional practice for personal relationships with other team members. • Acquire insights into basis for practice of other professions on team. • Establish a personal structure for teaching new members about one's profession and role on team.	• Practice active awareness of respectful communication with other team members. • Discuss controversies and problems with others. • Get to know and assimilate new members into teamwork processes.
Team	• Promote respect, truth telling, beneficence, and justice in relationships with other team members. • Address communication and conflict problems. • Develop understanding of differences in values, methods, and contributions of other team members. • Share responsibility for promoting team and accountability for its decisions and outcomes.	• Integrate professional knowledge with other team members. • Develop integrated patient problem definitions and a structure for assessment and care planning. • Promote and protect team as distinct structure.	• Develop ethic of open communication and dialogue. • Arrive on time for team meetings. • Develop and implement integrated patient care plans.

Organization	• Respect unique relationship between the team and the patient. • Understand basic principles of teamwork. • Provide sufficient resources for the team to accomplish its work and fulfill its mission.	• Provide sufficient resource foundation for team. • Establish evaluative structures for assessment of team's work.	• Support team development and function. • Appoint facilitator to address communication and ethics issues and mediate team conflicts.

Principles

Moral principles embody general guidelines for behavior based on established ethical concepts that are the foundation for developing and maintaining human relationships and communities. These principles are frequently employed in biomedical ethics as a way to understand and resolve ethical dilemmas in clinical practice. However, dilemmas may arise when principles conflict with each other, and the task becomes one of establishing their relative importance or ranking.

Individual Level

The individual level includes both personal and professional dimensions; the healthcare provider is both an individual person and a healthcare professional from a particular discipline. Certain norms, principles, and responsibilities guide each healthcare provider and reflect the individual's personal background as well as professional education. Some commonly invoked principles governing interpersonal relationships in healthcare settings are respect, truth-telling, beneficence, and justice. Most healthcare professions have established codes of ethics that emphasize the responsibility of the provider to honor patient autonomy and self-determination, to be honest in relationships, to be motivated by a wish to enhance well-being, and to promote fairness in healthcare resource distribution and decision making.

When thinking about the IHT, we can argue that the individual has the following obligations: (1) to develop competency in one's own discipline as the basis for mutual respect among the professions on the team, (2) to understand the norms and practice standards of the other professions on the team, and (3) to master the basic knowledge and skills required for effective teamwork. The foundation for these responsibilities is the need for the individual to master the individual professional and teamwork competencies required for effective collaborative practice.

Team Level

At this level, team members still retain their individual personal and professional guidelines for conduct, but added to them are new, higher-order, team-based expectations. Now situations arise that may bring members into conflict with their own or their profession's precepts, as well as those of the other team members. For example, a core set of values for team-based health care that has recently been articulated by the Institute of Medicine to guide the development of effective and high-functioning teams includes: (1) honesty in communication, (2) discipline in carrying out roles and responsibilities, (3) creativity in taking on new or emerging problems, (4) humility in relationships with other team members, and (5) curiosity in undertaking reflection in the pursuit of continuous improvement in team functioning.[9]

Importantly, IHT members have a responsibility to promote these principles in their relationships with each other. This requirement elevates responsibilities for team practice to the level of moral requirement, not personal preference or motivation. In addition, members have a mutual obligation to address communication problems and to constructively confront conflict that interferes with the team's ability to work effectively on solving complex clinical problems. Part of this duty is to develop a mutual understanding and integration of value differences among the health professions. Team members now have a set of relational and reciprocal requirements to learn about the other professions, how their contributions to improving patient care are related, and how to integrate different approaches to assessment and care plan development.

Finally, ethical concepts applied to the IHT increasingly emphasize the importance of shared responsibility and accountability of the healthcare team members, both for each other and for the decisions made by the team. This obligation includes the shared accountability of each member for the team's decisions and outcomes. Traditionally, the discussion of responsibility has focused on individuals as moral agents, not groups or teams. Recently, however, it has been argued that collectives can also be held accountable when that term is used to refer to a specific type of group—one whose members are unified or integrated in a particular manner.

Importantly, the argument for collective accountability hinges on the definition, level of function, and phase of development of the team. For example, the defined roles of different healthcare professionals on a team must be related to the patient care problem(s) at issue, as when the expertise of various health professionals is required to address the complex, multifaceted needs of an older adult. In addition, the level of integrated functioning of the IHT is critical for it to be termed a "collectivity." A multidisciplinary team—in which different professions offer their contributions in parallel or serial fashion—would not be considered a collective in the same sense that an IHT would because of the IHT's capacity for integrated dialogue.

However, even if the team serves as a collectivity and is jointly responsible for the outcomes of its actions (or inactions), members can still be held responsible individually for their behavior. Thus, in an ethical sense, members of an interprofessional team are responsible and accountable individually and collectively, creating a layered set of moral principles guiding their behavior.

Organizational Level

As mentioned at the beginning of this chapter, increasingly in the United States the provision of health care is occurring within a market economy dominated by the business model. In spite of recent calls that businesses and organizations articulate a clearly defined set of ethical values that guide them in a corporate vision and purpose, more and more the driving force in healthcare organizations is simply cost savings and profit making. These objectives run counter to the types of values that have traditionally governed interpersonal healthcare relationships at the levels of the individual and the team. Increasingly, the discourse of interprofessional teamwork is being co-opted by managers and investors. "Old" values such as providing care with compassion, treating employees with respect, and acting in a public spirit[10] are being replaced with the "new" values of economics. In fact, new books on healthcare teamwork increasingly employ the language of business and management in their discussion of the need for, and requirements of, interprofessional collaboration.

Structures

Structures are established patterns of thought and behavior within an organization for individual and collective practices related to IHTs. Research on ethical issues and teamwork has drawn attention to the importance of the social context within which moral dilemmas and the application of principles occur, the day-to-day environment in which providers work at the intersection of interpersonal, professional, organizational, and legal factors.[11] These structures may be either formal—based on established codes of practice and behavior that are codified into rules and regulations—or informal, occurring outside the boundaries of memoranda, meetings, and medical records.

Individual Level

As discussed in Chapter 4, healthcare professionals are socialized into traditional and expected modes of thought and patterns of behavior, including how individual patient problems are framed and addressed. Professional codes of ethics reinforce these cognitive and behavioral expectations for practitioners, and prescribe established frameworks for action that are congruent with a particular profession. An individual professional's contributions to teamwork are based on the quality of his or her training and understanding of the importance of his or her role in contributing to patient care on the IHT. Team members have a responsibility for developing standards of collaborative practice that form the basis for relationships with the other members of the team.

Team Level

As healthcare providers gain more experience in working together, a growing sense of loyalty to the joint practices and shared expectations that support the integrity and efficiency of the IHT should emerge. In addition, members have a responsibility for developing integrated patient assessment methods and associated care plans to ensure that their collaborative efforts are effective in meeting patients' needs. Related to this requirement, members of an IHT have an obligation to participate in the team dialogue and discourse, in order that their voices be heard in the definition of patient problems and the determination of solutions to them. Finally, members of the team have a responsibility for promoting and protecting the team as a distinct structure in the clinical setting in the face of challenges from within or without. In this respect, the team itself represents a distinctive structure for scaffolding effective and efficient patient care.

The development and refinement of a written set of team bylaws is a concrete example of how team members can jointly establish common rules and regulations governing their collaboration. The bylaws can specify guidelines for how meetings will be run, communication outside of meetings conducted, and basic expectations on individual behavior codified. When conflict arises, the structure of a set of bylaws can help teams address and, hopefully, resolve it.

Organizational Level

The focus of ethical mandates regarding teamwork at the level of the organization relate to the provision of sufficient resources to support the team in its ongoing development and maintenance and recognition when a team is in distress. This might include time for team meetings that is not billable and giving team managers time to manage the team. Short-term economic gain at the expense of teamwork effectiveness will undercut the team's ability to accomplish its mission.

Processes

Processes can be conceptualized as the content or activities that occur within the structures previously discussed. Structures are the frameworks, processes are the actual actions within them. The emphasis in procedural ethics is on the fairness of how problems are defined and solutions to them sought and implemented. As previously discussed in Chapter 4, in this process the quality of communication and the extent to which conflicts are identified and effectively addressed become critically important.

Individual Level

Procedural ethics requires that we treat other persons as "ends in themselves" rather than as "means to another end." In other words, we should not use other persons to achieve our own goals or objectives; rather, we need to treat them in a way that reinforces their own personal and professional worth, dignity, and respect. Team members should practice respectful communication with each other and openly discuss conflicts and controversies with other team members, including those with diverse levels of training. Talking about other team members behind their backs, secretly criticizing or discrediting the contributions of others on the team, and ganging up on certain members of the team are all examples of behaviors that procedural ethics would consider to be interprofessionally immoral.

Team Level

Teamwork requires a "procedural ethic" or process that emphasizes the importance of moral dialogue, discourse, and debate. This includes communication regarding the different value orientations acquired by different professionals in their educational socialization. Relevant to teamwork is Moody's argument for a "communicative ethic" based on deliberation and negotiation and leading to improved communication, clarification, and consensus-building in addressing the complex situations in which conflicts between ethical principles lead to difficult moral dilemmas.[12]

In addition, David Thomasma has characterized the development of such a procedural ethic on teams as the "moral education of interdisciplinary teams" to "bring about a concert of moral interests within a team."[13] IHTs need to devote time and resources to designing their teamwork process, and a procedural ethic becomes a guideline for developing a shared and unified moral climate in which teamwork dialogue and discourse are promoted and protected.

Organizational Level

Similar to structural factors, procedurally the organization must actively support the team in developing its internal processes for ensuring communication, dealing with conflict, and addressing ethical concerns that may arise in the team itself. In addition, the organization and the team need to have communication processes ensuring that both parties are aware of the issues affecting their relationship. This is an important level that is often overlooked in the literature on IHTs.

As mentioned at the beginning of this chapter, ethical issues in health care arise in the relationships that providers have with their patients as well as with each other. Our next focus in this chapter, then, will be on how professional values affect those patient relationships at a basic level. Chapter 4 explored how communication and conflict issues in teamwork involve an understanding of the different values that characterize the process of becoming a healthcare professional, of being socialized into the role of physician, nurse, or social worker. These value differences affect the ways in which providers communicate with their patients and understand issues involving their lives. Similarly, they make a major difference in patterns of clinical practice, affecting elements related to how practitioners define problems, grapple with issues involving quality of life, and practice collaborative decision making.

Case Study, Take 3: Mr. Robert Crane

The case study introduced earlier involves an IHT assessment of Mr. Crane's health issues. Thus, the nurse, physician, and social worker (and the other health professionals available to join the team as needed) have a unique set of ethical responsibilities based on the principles, structures, and processes discussed in the framework.

The Geriatrics Assessment and Care Planning Team at Shady Grove Hospital has been working together for nearly three years. Its primary members are Ms. Debbie Espinoza, a clinical nurse specialist; Dr. Marilyn Gettes, a geriatrician; and Mr. Ying Sun, the social worker. When they first started their work together, it took them a while to learn about each other's backgrounds and areas of training and competence, as well as their clinical expertise and skills in working with older adults. Importantly, they had to learn about the different values that guided their personal lives and professional practice, as well as to feel comfortable in trusting each other in performing their roles and responsibilities on the IHT.

After a somewhat rocky start, due to the fact that none of them had had any experience in working on a team, they were able to make a collective commitment to improving their communication among themselves and their ability to address conflict when it arose in team meetings or during assessments. The hospital CEO was supportive of their work and assisted in identifying teamwork training resources and paying for continuing educational programs that provided them with some basic teamwork skills. Because of the challenging complexity of many of their geriatrics cases, they have had to pull together as a team and to rely on each other's expertise in addressing their patients' problems. Now, they feel a real strength in "having the team behind them" when they come to a consensus and make difficult decisions about complex cases.

By the time Mr. Crane came into the clinic for his assessment, the team members felt a high degree of loyalty to the IHT and each other. They had worked hard to set up structures and processes to govern their collaborative work. For example, they had developed a set of teamwork bylaws that were periodically updated to reflect new insights and issues. When interpersonal conflicts among them started becoming a problem, they brought in an outside consultant to help them work through these challenges. The struggles to deal with these problems have made them even more committed to the team and each other. When faced with cases such as Mr. Crane's, they work hard to come to a collective decision that includes input from each member of the team, respecting differences that may still exist.

After individually gathering data on Mr. Crane with nursing, medical, and social work assessments, the team came together to discuss their findings and develop a care plan that would simultaneously take into account his areas of need, as well as his strengths and resources. The team decided it was important to respect his autonomy and wish to remain at home, while at the same time recognizing that he was facing some risks by staying there. Assessments revealed some minor cognitive impairment, though not sufficient to compromise his stated commitment to living on his own. Working with his daughter, the team was able to get him to accept some homemaking assistance for cooking and housekeeping, with a visiting nurse coming once a week for basic health monitoring. Any change in his condition would trigger a follow-up from the team, including a possible home visit by the nurse and the social worker. The team felt that this solution provided a good balance between respecting Mr. Crane's autonomy and wishes to stay in his own home, and recognizing his daughter's concern about his safety and the avoidance of unnecessary risks.

Summary

Ethical issues in health care are often challenging, especially so when set against the backdrop of IHT practice; this chapter has presented the different dimensions of ethical issues in IHTs. These are both horizontal and vertical. Each member of the team has horizontal responsibilities toward other professionals on the team, based on an understanding of their own unique values and those of the other professionals on the IHT. In addition, vertical responsibilities include relationships with patients on the one hand, and with administrators within the healthcare organization on the other. These relationships are heavily influenced by professional codes of conduct and differ among the different professions on the team. They include the dimensions of principles, structures, and processes. These factors expand our traditional ethical thinking, which is usually focused on principles, to dimensions of professional practice that are unique to teamwork settings and include the rules, roles, and responsibilities of being an IHT member.

The development of a proposed framework for conceptualizing ethical issues arising from interprofessional teamwork, and its application to a clinical case study, can help to define and lay out the basic structure of the field of interprofessional ethics. The following set of conclusions is intended to summarize the implications of this work and provide a set of principles guiding future developments in this emerging area.

Importance of a Framework

Just as the field of interprofessional education and practice is beginning to recognize the need for greater conceptual clarity and theoretical sophistication, so too do we need to develop a better understanding of the complex and multifaceted ethical issues that inevitably arise in IHTs. The development of a framework must be applicable to a wide array of teamwork contexts and settings—whether primary, acute, or long-term care—and incorporate the key elements found in the literature and clinical practice of principles, structures, and processes. An examination of these factors at the levels of the individual, the team, and the organization reveals particular areas of congruence and conflict at the interface between the professional and the patient and among the professionals on the team.

Interprofessional Ethics Discourse

We also need to recognize that furthering the discourse on interprofessional ethics is itself essential. Characterizing issues in IHTs as ethical ones, as concerns that raise significant normative questions, elevates the discussion of teamwork issues to a new plane of moral discourse. Most of the IHT literature has historically emphasized group process concepts and models, based on sociology and psychology. Introducing insights from philosophy and ethics has the potential to provide important new dimensions that will simultaneously improve patient care and teamwork effectiveness and efficiency. By invoking the language of rights and responsibilities, we have added a new dimension to the discussion on teamwork and interprofessional collaboration. As new calls are made to focus on the incorporation of values into teamwork training to achieve necessary competencies for collaborative practice, it is important that there be sustained attention to developing a theoretical foundation for teaching this knowledge and skills base in the different health professions.

Interprofessional Ethics as an Emerging Field

With the establishment of a basic structure and the initial development of a language for the discourse of interprofessional ethics, we can begin to recognize the unique moral dilemmas arising from collaborative teamwork in a healthcare setting. New moral issues will be identified as recommendations for expanded teamwork practice increase in number and complexity, and the reliance on collaboration across care professions and within varied settings increases. These concerns are qualitatively different from those that are typically addressed within the biomedical ethics frameworks currently available. Changing patterns of healthcare practice often create new moral dilemmas and ethical concerns, and now is time to embrace these interprofessional issues and develop new ways of addressing them.

This need is particularly acute at the interface between interprofessional education and practice, the point of contact between educators and practitioners. Educators must be aware of the unique demands of teamwork practice so that they can adequately prepare professionals for the normative demands introduced by collaboration in addressing the often complex needs of challenging patients, whether in the fields of geriatrics, palliative care, developmental disabilities, or mental health. These settings are often the most fraught with moral dilemmas, difficulties, and disparities.

For example, IHTs working with older adults with multiple, chronic health conditions; patients at the end of life who are facing difficult decisions about the types of care they want to receive; children or adults with developmental disabilities that make competency questionable and decision making challenging; and persons with mental health problems that pose unique challenges to continuity of care between acute and community-based settings—all these IHTs face situations every day that call for reflection on ethical principles and the establishment of structures and processes helping to guide their decision making.

In addition, and as discussed at the beginning of this chapter, the growing intrusion of a business model—with its attendant emphases on cost savings and profit making—into health care, in general, and IHTs, in particular, promises to replace the traditional ethical values and moral principles we associate with providing care with economic values and the management language of cost, profit, and efficiency. This development is particularly significant as it may signal a retreat from a primary focus on quality of care and the provision of resources necessary to promote it, to a reduction in education and professional development for the sake of concern about "the bottom line." This situation would have a dramatic and negative effect on interprofessional education and practice.

It has been our goal in this chapter to raise the visibility of these issues to help move the field of interprofessional education and practice forward in a new and exciting direction—that of interprofessional ethics. The future direction of health care promises to make these issues increasingly relevant and important.

Questions for Discussion

1. What are some of the ethical challenges you have encountered while working on IHTs? What were the underlying causes of these conflicts?
2. How might you use the framework of "principles, structures, and processes" to help understand the types of dilemmas found in teamwork practice? Is this approach helpful? What are its strengths and weaknesses?

3. Do you think IHTs require a whole "new" type of ethical thinking based on the complexity of teamwork and all that it entails, or can we just use the "old" type of thinking based on the moral guidelines of individual professions and tweak it to fit collaborative practice?

4. How can we best educate team members to identify and address the unique ethical issues that arise in teamwork practice?

10

Theory in Interprofessional Education: There Is Nothing So Practical as a Good Theory[*]

There is nothing so practical as a good theory.

—Kurt Lewin[1]

We don't see things as they are; we see things as we are.

—Anaïs Nin[2]

The real voyage of discovery consists not in seeking new landscapes, but in having new eyes.

—Marcel Proust[3]

Introduction

For many healthcare providers and even some educators and researchers, the last thing they would like to think about is theory. Let's just say that theory has a mixed reputation, and it seems to be frequently

---

[*] Parts of this chapter are based on two previous publications: Clark, P. G. (2006). What would a theory of interprofessional education look like? Some suggestions for developing a theoretical framework for teamwork training. *Journal of Interprofessional Care, 20*: 577–589; and Clark, P. G. (2009). Reflecting on reflection in interprofessional education: Implications for theory and practice. *Journal of Interprofessional Care, 23*: 213–223.

overlooked in the hustle and bustle of everyday work. The stereotype of people interested in theory is the isolated and reclusive academic hermit living in the ivory tower who seldom has to come down and deal with real-world issues in the everyday messiness of life.

However, it is also true that the importance of theory increases in proportion to the stage of development of a new discipline or profession. As a field grows in maturity, those interested in it begin to recognize the need for a stronger conceptual or theoretical foundation for supporting teaching and developing research. So it is with the field of interprofessional education (IPE), which has evolved sufficiently to embrace the concept that there is now "nothing so practical" or, we might add, "so essential," as a good theory or set of theories. Until recently, much of the literature in IPE has been descriptive, anecdotal, or atheoretical, and there is now clearly the need for a more sustained development of its theoretical foundation. Such a framework certainly can be useful in developing programs and courses in the educational setting; but, perhaps more importantly, it is essential in designing research and evaluation projects that can assess the impacts and outcomes of educational interventions. For example, a report from the Institute of Medicine has called for more research on measuring the impact of IPE on collaborative practice and patient outcomes.[4]

The purpose of this chapter is to propose an outline of what might be some of the critical components of a theoretical framework for IPE, and, in particular, how they might collectively construct a comprehensive theory to direct the development of effective educational programs to train healthcare professions students and providers in the essentials of IHTs. Even though we may fall short of a truly comprehensive "theory of everything IPE" in this effort, we may still attain an adequate framework to provide guidance for educational and research program development. In many ways, just raising the awareness of the importance of theory is a step in the right direction for promoting its use in IPE.

In this chapter, we start with an overview of why theory is important, and then proceed to discuss the following elements: (1) cooperative, collaborative, or social learning, (2) experiential learning, (3) the epistemology and ontology of interprofessional inquiry, and (4) reflection and the reflective practitioner.

Definition and Role of Theory in IPE

Theory may be defined most simply as "the construction of explicit explanations in accounting for empirical findings."[5] The practicality of theory is related to its ability to integrate and explain knowledge, predict what is not yet observed or known, and develop interventions to solve problems. Instructional or research-related work that is conducted without a strong theoretical basis is like a "floating skyscraper" without a solid foundation upon which to build. It may seem impressive, but until such an effort is brought down to earth and rooted in a firm theoretical tradition, its ability to undergird program development or evaluation is extremely limited.

One application of theory to IPE is to support basic instructional practice, where the following questions need to be answered: (1) what does it mean to "learn to do" interprofessional teamwork? and (2) how can educators facilitate achieving these instructional outcomes? In addressing these needs, IPE theory should (1) identify and describe major concepts to guide the design of course and curricular structures and processes, (2) specify learning objectives and effective methods to achieve them, (3) suggest appropriate roles for students and teachers, and (4) facilitate the measurement of program impacts and outcomes for students or participants.

A second, and no less important, application of theory in IPE is to support research. Much research in this area has been atheoretical and not conducted with the guidance of a conceptual framework. This need applies to both basic research into the kinds of outcomes that can be achieved by IPE and applied research into designing the most effective strategies for how to achieve these outcomes. As the field of IPE moves forward with more research and graduate-level program development, it will need a continued effort to propose and refine theoretical frameworks to guide and sustain it. This development is a critical aspect of the further evolution of IPE as a distinct academic field worthy of investigation and research.

IPE now needs to consider how to construct a coherent theoretical framework for use in articulating the structures and describing the processes for both educators and researchers. Making theory more explicit "encourages systematic, disciplined, and critical thinking [and] informs decisions and generates propositions which can be tested."[6] In this sense, theory aids in meeting the interrelated goals of effective instruction and educational research.

The next section of this chapter lays out a suggested framework for the facets and factors related to the development of IPE theory.

Some Components of IPE Theory

A commonly used definition of IPE is "occasions when two or more professions learn with, from, and about each other to improve collaboration and the quality of care."[7] This seemingly simple definition suggests some major features of IPE: (1) the students or professionals are in a group setting where they learn in collaboration with each other; (2) participants also learn from each other in the sense that education has an experiential basis; in other words, learning occurs by doing; and (3) learners gain insights into each other's background, education, and roles in health care. This type of learning has several interrelated theoretical components, as will be made apparent in the discussion that follows.

Cooperative, Collaborative, or Social Learning

As already discussed, a primary foundation for IPE is cooperative, collaborative, or social learning. By this definition we mean group-based learning, in contrast with the individualistic approach that typically predominates more generally in higher education. Instead of the model in which the student learns the knowledge that is considered important from the instructor, and then is assessed using individualized tests, the group model emphasizes the social aspects of learning that follow more closely real-world settings, in which learning occurs in interaction with others. In particular, educators have noted that the kinds of knowledge and skills needed by healthcare professionals to work together in teams are often those acquired by using problem- or case-based methods that require students to work collaboratively in solving complex or multifaceted problems.

Three characteristics of this model of learning have major implications for IPE. First, rather than knowledge being "out there" to be learned as if it were a disembodied entity to be deposited into students' brains, knowledge in IPE is created in the interactions and interrelationships among the members of the group. The social exchanges among the members are the ground upon which knowledge grows and evolves. The students or participants learn about each other's professional backgrounds, training, and perspectives, and they acquire the basic skills of teamwork related to leadership, communication, and conflict. For example, in our experience students frequently do not know how providers in the other health professions are educated, what they study, or how they gain clinical experience. They often do not understand the scopes of practice of other professionals, or where there are areas of overlap or separation. In courses or workshops we have taught, we often find that participants are interested in learning more about the education and backgrounds of different professions represented in the group.

As the Canadian communication theorist, Marshall McLuhan, observed, "the medium is the message," meaning that the process of learning is really the learning itself. In a similar vein, John Dewey, the great American philosopher of education, noted that you cannot teach someone the skills they need to learn from experience, but you can direct them in the way they need to go to learn them. This model of education is less about the instructor being the "sage on the stage," and more the teacher as the "coach on the playing field."

Second, knowledge learned in this way is closely related to the formation of professional or clinical judgment, which is more closely linked to the interrelationships among people than between people and objects. Students have the opportunity to correct each other's biases and question false assumptions, thereby gaining experience in interactions that promote better care in actual clinical settings for their future work as professionals. Insofar as some of the current support for IHTs stems from concerns about patient safety in the healthcare system, this theoretical basis suggests an important outcome of teamwork is the prevention of mistakes based on unquestioned assumptions and reluctance to challenge the positions or recommendations of other professionals. Indeed, some approaches to IHT education teach members how to use methods originally developed in aviation safety to call for "time out" in clinical situations to question something that does not seem right.

Third, IPE must be based on the recognition that all knowledge in the professions is socially constructed. The basic cognitive structures of a discipline (to be discussed in more detail below) are acquired in communities of practice with faculty, students, and peers who share the same socialization process and worldview. Becoming a professional means acquiring the same patterns of thought and behavior as others in the same profession. For example, in higher education settings, we cluster and cloister health professions students in their own separate courses and academic programs, often physically located in different buildings and locations on campus. Importantly, IPE provides an opportunity for students to see the world through eyes different from their own, as the quotation from Marcel Proust at the beginning of this chapter suggests. This experience of "decentering," of getting out of your own frame of reference and becoming aware of viewpoints different from one's own, is an essential outcome of IPE experiences.[8]

Experiential Learning

If collaborative learning creates the structure for IPE, then experiential learning provides the process. In this context, learning is dependent on the experience of IPE itself and leads to the acquisition of insights and skills by the participants. As discussed earlier, interprofessional teamwork is best conceived of as something to be learned by actually doing it, rather than by reading a book or discussing it in a classroom. Moreover, as the educational theorist David Kolb[9] has suggested, experiential learning is based on a cycle of distinct states: feeling, watching, thinking, and doing.

According to experiential learning theory, distinct styles of learning exist along two axes: (1) concrete experience (CE)—"feeling"—versus abstract conceptualization (AC)—"thinking," and (2) active experimentation (AE)—"doing"—versus reflective observation (RO)—"watching." Learning as a process based on experience must include all these elements: learners must participate in new experiences (CE), observe and reflect on these experiences from different perspectives (RO), develop concepts that integrate their observations into logical theories (AC), and then use these theories to make decisions and solve problems (AE).

Because IPE and interprofessional practice (IPP) have often been linked to efforts to improve the quality of health care, it is interesting to note that methods of continuous quality improvement (CQI) use a similar approach called PDSA cycles—Plan (P), Do (D), Study (S), and Act (A). In the clinical context, this method involves planning to implement an intervention focused on solving a particular problem, doing it, collecting data or studying whether it was effective, and acting again to refine the intervention—all in a continuous cycle of quality improvement.

Practically speaking, students learning to work as an interprofessional team should expect to work collaboratively either in real clinical settings, in patient simulation labs, or on problem-based case studies that mimic real-world situations. In such contexts, students must learn to balance the need for profession-specific knowledge and skills with those essential for working together as a team. Students need to have sufficient education that they know the basics of their own profession and how to play their own, unique role on the team; on the other hand, they cannot be so "set in their (professional) ways" that they cannot or will not be open to learning about others' roles and areas of knowledge and expertise. Thus, the timing of the IPE experience is important to maximize its impact on the individual professional-in-training.

Finally, a particularly critical dimension of IPE, and one that is part of the learning cycle, is reflection. It is important that specific instructional methods of encouraging reflection are integrated into the learning experience. This topic will be discussed in more detail later in this chapter.

Epistemology and Ontology of Interprofessional Inquiry

Another critical component of IPE is the recognition that different health professions "see the world not as it is, but as they are," as the quotation from Anaïs Nin at the beginning of this chapter suggests. Who we are depends on our understanding of both knowledge and values. These two aspects of professional identity shape our sense of self as a professional, how we relate to the patient, and the ways in which we interact with other healthcare providers. This topic was also discussed in Chapter 4.

Epistemology, the philosophical study or theory of knowledge, focuses on the origin, nature, limits, methods, and justification of knowledge—how we understand, acquire, process, and share information. It recognizes the fact that each health profession is based on the mastery and utilization of distinct types of expert information. Indeed, different professions have been developed as they have increasingly defined and defended the acquisition and application of their specific type of knowledge. Petrie[10] has termed the knowledge foundation of each profession its *cognitive map*, which includes its basic concepts, modes of inquiry, problem definitions, observational categories, representational techniques, standards of proof, types of explanation, and general ideas of what represents a discipline. The cognitive map is a virtual one that helps each professional in a specific discipline to "see the same thing when they look at the same thing," a lens acquired in the process of professional socialization that ensures a uniform approach to the patient and similarity in assessing problems and developing care plans.

Beyond epistemology, however, is another domain of professional practice, one that focuses on values, the processing of value-relevant information, and the framing of moral dilemmas. Analogous to its cognitive map, each profession also has its own normative map, which includes basic values, modes of moral reasoning, and methods for resolving ethical dilemmas. Taken together, these elements constitute the "ontological" component of professional identity, that related to who one is as a professional (ontology is the philosophical study or theory of the nature of being). As discussed in Chapter 4, values make up an important part of our identity as a professional, resulting from the internalization of norms, standards, and meanings of a profession. In addition, different professionals have differing codes of ethics and moral standards for practice into which they are socialized as students and practitioners.[11, 12]

In fact, the whole process of socialization to become a professional involves the acquisition of particular traditions, customs, and practices;

knowledge, beliefs, morals, and rules of conduct; and linguistic and symbolic forms of communication and the meanings they share that are associated with the practice of that particular profession.[13] This process creates a professional who thinks and behaves differently from others. As explored in Chapter 4, professional identity or self-concept is based on the narratives or stories that we tell about ourselves as professionals, and they serve as the basis for how we relate both to patients and to other healthcare providers.

The implications of cognitive and normative maps for IPE are far-reaching. First of all, members of the healthcare team must become aware of their own maps, to gain insight into the frameworks they use to make sense of the world as seen through the eyes of their own profession. Second, they must learn about the maps of the other professionals on the team, and start appreciating how their interaction with the world is different. Importantly, these understandings should culminate in the members of a team recognizing that all these perspectives are important to the IHT in addressing the whole patient and his or her complex needs and problems. This process is a key aspect of students learning about each other, their education and training, how they think, and the ways in which they approach the patient.

This second dimension of teamwork learning requires the acquisition of interpretive knowledge, the ability of one professional to understand the observational categories, meanings, judgments, and recommendations of another professional. For example, Lattuca[14] suggests that this situation requires the borrowing or appropriation of the tools of another discipline in one's own work—based on the previously discussed concept of decentering, of becoming aware of viewpoints different from one's own and how they may help frame a patient's problem or issue to provide more insight and understanding. This concept is related to the notion of "metacognitive competence," in which an individual is simultaneously able to think both about their own thinking and that of others.[15]

For example, we have a nursing colleague, Pat, who was doing a presentation in a workshop on geriatric assessment and talking about how a nurse would approach a patient. Then, she stopped, and without missing a beat, stepped to the other side of the podium and said, "Now here's how John (our physician colleague) would approach this problem." After explaining how a geriatrician would think and behave, she stepped back to her original side of the podium and stated, "Now, I'm back as Pat and am a nurse again." This ability to toggle back and forth between two different professions is a good example of interpretive knowledge at work.

A metaphor for this use and mastery of differing cognitive and normative maps of different professions is that of "tool kit." Just as a carpenter, plumber, or electrician has their own tool kit associated with their work and trade, consisting of the tools they have learned to use skillfully, so too does each healthcare professional have his or her own type of knowledge, skills, values, and behaviors associated with competent clinical practice. Using a tool from a different tradesperson (such as an electrician using a saw or a hammer when installing wires) does not make them that other profession, but it may help them to do their work more efficiently or effectively.

So, too, a healthcare professional may utilize a tool from another professional to assess a patient's needs more effectively and to provide a more appropriate strategy for addressing them. Moreover, each professional must recognize the limits of their own abilities and tools when approaching a complex situation or a difficult patient and know when the knowledge and skills of another, different professional are needed to provide high quality patient care. To extend our earlier metaphor, the electrician will need to know when to call in a carpenter to perform the work that is necessary for a high-quality result.

Reflection and the Reflective Practitioner

Reflection has emerged as a key concept in educational theory and learning, especially in the health professions. It is typically associated not only with profession-specific education, but also with respect to teamwork learning and practice. As discussed earlier, it is a critical component of the learning cycle in general[16] and with regard to IPE specifically.[17] Not surprisingly, the term *reflection* has multiple meanings. First, it relates to learning and the (re)presentation of learning, of thinking about something in more detail; second, it suggests a purpose, goal, or outcome; and third, reflection involves higher-order mental processes. In this final context, for example, it may mean relying on more complicated mental processing of issues or problems for which there is no easy solution. This "critical thinking" aspect of the meaning may require stepping back from a situation to (re)view it.

Importantly for IPE, clarity on the level of reflection is important. Wackerhausen,[18] for example, differentiates between "primary" and "secondary" reflection. Primary, or first-order, reflection is too closely allied with one's own personal and professional views and perspectives, with one's own way of seeing the world. What is needed for transformative

IPE learning is secondary or second-order reflection that requires stepping back from oneself and professional perspective to consider one's own self and others. This "perspective transformation" or critical reflection is akin to the concept of decentering discussed earlier. Achieving the goal of metacognitive competence requires "thinking about one's own thinking."

We may extend this concept to reflection and consider being able to "reflect on one's own reflection" or "meta-reflection" as an example of the kinds of processes needed for effective IPE experiences. This distinction is related to our earlier discussion about interpretive knowledge and the professional tool kit, of learning about how other professions see the world and beginning to use their perspectives in one's own thinking about the patient and patient care. Both deal with perspective shift or transformation, and the ability to consider or reflect simultaneously on one's own and other's ways of being and seeing.

Reflection as an ability, particularly at the higher or secondary level, seems to vary by profession. Different professionals seem to have more or less ability to be reflective, depending on their socialization and education. For example, in our work with IPE and IPP, we have noted that nursing and social work students seem to be more comfortable with reflection than those from medicine, pharmacy, and physical therapy. Students from nursing and social work are more likely to have had written assignments requiring some type of reflection or an experiential or clinical placement upon which they have had to practice reflection. This observation is consistent with Kolb's[19] work, which suggests that nursing and social work are more "divergent" professions that emphasize concrete experience and reflective observation, whereas the more medically oriented professions are more "convergent" and rely more on abstract conceptualization and active experimentation.

More practically, the concept of reflection is also used by Schön[20] in his work on educating the reflective practitioner, who is that professional trained in both the scientific dimensions of practice—the technical knowledge and skills of that profession—and the so-called artistic elements—those related to the ability to grapple with the gray or indeterminate areas of practice. These are the situations encountered in which moral ambiguity, value conflicts, and ethical dilemmas are to be found.

For Schön, technical rationality is the epistemology of professional practice, when practitioners use scientifically selected means to solve particular problems. In contrast, the ontology of professional practice involves framing the specific issues to be addressed and determining the appropriate directions for action to be taken. Particularly relevant to IPE, the framing of a problem requires an understanding of how different pro-fessions have differing perspectives on what it is and how to solve it. In addition, and as discussed earlier, this ability includes the recognition of the limits of one's own type of knowledge and skill set, and when to rely on those of other professionals.

Thus, Schön's theory supports the importance of IPE in the develop-ment of sound clinical judgment on the part of healthcare professionals by seeing the patient through the lenses of other providers. Perhaps we can extend the metaphor of the "reflective practitioner" to that of the "reflective team member" who is constantly considering his or her own knowledge and skills, that of other professionals, and how the two are interrelated in a complex and complementary fashion. This insight sug-gests that one of the goals of IHT development is to achieve this level of personal and professional development among all the members of the team.

A Concrete Example of Theoretical Concepts in Practice

A concrete example of an actual IPE course may serve to illustrate how specific components of theory may be used in the development of require-ments and assignments. This example will emphasize the use of reflection and student work that is based on it.

Course Goals and Objectives

For over 30 years, an elective course on interprofessional teamwork has been taught at the University of Rhode Island. Its objectives are to:

1. Learn the basic knowledge necessary for understanding the essential dimensions of teamwork practice, including communication, conflict, leadership, role negotiation, and advocacy.
2. Acquire basic understanding of major concepts, principles, and theories of teamwork as they relate to interprofessional collaboration in health care, human service, and education settings.
3. Apply the basic knowledge of teamwork to real-world healthcare and human service contexts where collaboration is essential to addressing prob-lems and improving the quality of care and of life.
4. Develop specific skills, abilities, and attitudes important for working with teams of healthcare and human service professionals.
5. Improve oral and written communication skills, as well as reflective prac-tice, in working with other professionals.

The course typically recruits six to eight advanced undergraduate and graduate students from the health and social care professions—including nursing, social work, pharmacy, medicine, nutrition, dental hygiene, and counseling—who are interested in learning more about health and social care teamwork.[21] It combines (1) a weekly seminar based on readings and discussion on teamwork theory dealing with such topics as communication, conflict, and leadership, with (2) problem-based learning (PBL) cases in which the students collaborate in small groups to work on patient/client assessment and care plan development.

Reflection Assignments

The central activity and learning context for the students is their small group work on the PBL cases, which is based on the principles of collaborative or cooperative and experiential learning discussed previously. While the weekly readings provide a conceptual structure for this experience, the actual learning occurs in the collaborative or cooperative experiential setting of these groups. Importantly, and in addition, reflection is a required and essential element of the course,[22] built upon two major assignments.

Journal

First, the students are required to keep a journal of their interactions and experiences, using a prescribed format that encourages them to make connections between teamwork theory and practice. In particular, the notes in the journal are constructed around key elements of the learning cycle. The journal represents an ongoing educational story or narrative for each student, constructed around their own internal dialogue and that between themselves and the other students. It encourages the participants to reflect on their own experiences and to recast, reinterpret, and reinforce their emerging ideas and insights. Requiring that the journal be written is a key component of its importance and impact, as it allows students to see how they have changed over the course of the semester and charts their development as a team member.

The importance of journaling for students in my IPE course is captured in the following statements from their coursework:

- "I learned that the journal served as a way to document our individual growth. When I wrote in my journal, it forced me to reflect back on the events, feelings, encounters, and interpretations that I experienced. I was able to attempt to make sense of them and analyze different approaches to handling these different events . . . I began to try to look at situations from the point of view that the other people may have had. I enjoyed looking back at my journal from the entire semester; I thought about where I came from, and where I have now come."

- "Journaling is the class, it is the teacher of the course . . . It forces thoughts to the forefront. If the thoughts were not written down, the observer may doubt their importance, and push them to the back of the mind . . . When forced to look at these thoughts and thought processes, one begins to learn from them. The knowledge gained from the observation and study of one experience leads to experimentation with alternative solutions the next time that situation arises. Ultimately, this can lead to the growth of the team."
- "The process of journaling became a tremendous source of insight for me throughout the semester. It ultimately enriched my academic and team experience, giving 'life' and meaning to many of those thoughts [to which] I would ordinarily have paid little attention. Journaling also facilitated my learning process by enabling me to connect theory with actual practice and experience."

Reflection Papers

Second, the participants complete two short three- to four-page reflection papers that are based on their journals and expand their thinking about the implications for themselves as professionals and for their team as a group. These papers allow them to expand their thinking on issues and patterns that are based on the notes in their journal, often topics related to the course themes of communication, conflict, and leadership. The reflection papers promote secondary reflection, with the student reflecting on their primary reflection captured in their journals. This additional level of reflection encourages the kind of "reflection on reflection" or meta-reflection described in the earlier theoretical discussion.

Learning outcomes for the students suggest deeper insight and understanding, as captured in the following observations:

- "Although I have been keeping a journal frequently through the semester, I never realized how strong a team was until I wrote my reflection paper. The paper helped organize my thoughts and made it very clear to me that there is a tremendous power in an interprofessional team."
- "In general, the reflection papers were another worthwhile portion [of the course] due to the fact that they made you think deeper about certain topics that you made note of in your journal. It was not always easy to reflect

on certain matters, but in the process of actually sitting down and thinking about certain team-related issues I was able to better understand a lot of the course concepts. My reflection papers were where I made the majority of my conclusions regarding the course and how it could be applied to actual situations."

These comments suggest that the papers provide an enhancement of the reflective process through an additional and expanded opportunity for the students to delve more deeply into the observational and thought processes represented in their journals, and to recognize patterns of growth and development in the experiences of the course over time.

Reflections on Reflection

This course and the assignments based on the importance of reflection as a key to transformative IPE outcomes provide an important example of how components of IPE theory can guide the development of educational programs and their requirements. In this case, reflection is an important method of achieving insights into the meaning of teamwork and how the students understand the requirements of interprofessional practice. Based on key elements of experiential learning theory, reflection as a concept can provide the foundation for the development and utilization of specific assignments to promote it as a key skill in learning how to practice on IHTs.

Implications of Theory for IPE

The implications of these four key elements or aspects of a theoretical foundation for IPE are important for the development of courses or programs, and also for their evaluation or assessment of learning outcomes. Overall, the intent of this chapter has been to demonstrate that the conceptual or theoretical components of IPE can be embedded in practical educational approaches, activities, and assignments.

IPE as a Social Process of Collaborative and Experiential Learning

Social relationships are the core of the IPE learning process, and they are best developed in the context of cooperative or collaborative learning with a practical or experiential "hands on" approach utilizing real-world or clinical case studies and applications. In this process, the students learn "with, from, and about" each other and master the essential skill set needed for collaborative practice. Such learning takes time and effort, and may best be conceptualized as a developmental process rather than a one-time exposure to IPE concepts.

In this regard, health professions students need to be socialized in two parallel tracks: (1) one for their own profession, and (2) one for working with other professions on the team. To use our earlier metaphor of "tool kit," they need to develop their own profession's tool kit and that of the team member or player. This process may require the development of a graded set of experiences or modules, from basic to advanced, over the course of an academic or continuing education program. In addition, it may need "scaffolded instruction," in which the emerging mastery of the IPE skill set requires multiple structures and opportunities for learning IHT practice until the necessary degree of mastery has been achieved.

Epistemology and Ontology, Facts and Values

Both the epistemology and the ontology of professional practice occur as themes in the theoretical foundation of IPE. A major objective must be the achievement of understanding both the cognitive and the normative bases of one's own profession and those of others on the team. Decentering is the process for achieving this outcome, one that requires getting out of one's own profession's perspective and inside that of others. As educators, we must empower our students to ask the following questions: (1) who am I (my own profession) and what do I know? (2) who are the others (the other professions on the team) and what do they know?, and (3) who are we collectively as a team and what do we know? These questions can lead to the assessment of learning outcomes in educational programs; in clinical settings, their achievement can be facilitated by the development of such methods as a common assessment methodology and a unified care plan in which the patient's problem is defined in a way that all professions can contribute to its solution.

In this regard, an expanded definition of a teamwork "tool kit" can be offered, in contrast to the professional one that is identified solely with the domain of each provider. The interprofessional tool kit consists of the ability to use a set of group skills, including communication methods, leadership roles, role negotiation, conflict management, problem solving, and decision making. The mastery of the tools in this kit requires parallel socialization into the collaborative methods described earlier and can, similar to the acquisition of a specific profession's knowledge and skills, be assessed and measured as educational outcomes.

Importance of Reflection

If IPE is to be truly transformative, it must incorporate higher-order reflection in its social and collaborative processes. In this regard, reflection becomes a key process for learning that builds on the cooperative and collaborative learning and experiential basis of IPE. One must simultaneously step outside of one's own professional perspective and into those of other providers, an interpersonal dimension. In addition, however, IPE must also involve an intrapersonal element as well, in which the student achieves a level of introspection into him- or herself and what it means to be a member of a specific profession.

For example, we have had students tell us that they did not really know themselves and the essence of what it means to be their profession until they participated in interprofessional learning experiences in which they learned about others from different backgrounds. As the Chinese philosopher Lao Tzu observed, "He who knows others is wise: he who knows himself is enlightened."[23] Because of its central importance to transformative learning, specific methods to encourage reflection must be built into IPE courses and programs.[24]

Implications for Student and Faculty Roles

IPE calls into question many of the fundamental methods and means of standard educational practice. Because of its radical nature, genuine IPE learning may not fit well into existing academic structures or programs. It is seldom a required experience for a health professions degree and is often difficult to fit logistically into an existing set of degree requirements. Teamwork learning is process-based and dependent on the experience of students working together in groups. The required knowledge and skills are learned through the actual process, and the students learn as much from each other about their different professional roles, backgrounds, and training as they do from the instructor.

In a fundamental way, the students need to learn that IPE is about the journey itself, not the outcome or the destination. As discussed earlier, this insight influences how we see the roles of students and faculty. Students teach each other and the experience provides the education, not the faculty member. Faculty can model effective teamwork behavior, serve as a resource to address problems as they arise, and monitor and guide student progress through the learning experience.

Beyond traditional academic programs for students, we also need to develop innovative and comprehensive continuing education programs for providers who did not receive teamwork training as part of their initial health professions education. The challenge for these types of programs is to build in both foundational knowledge and skills development and ongoing support for professionals who continue to work collaboratively in the clinical or practice setting. The achievement of these goals may require nontraditional educational methods, such as online or Web-based experiences and instruction.

Summary

Theory in IPE can be as helpful in framing and assessing learning outcomes as it is in developing actual instructional programs. Thus, it has equally important roles in the development of educational experiences and in the research increasingly needed to assess their impacts and measure their effectiveness. The field of IPE has developed to a point at which theory will be increasingly important, and it has been the goal of this chapter to demonstrate that, indeed, "there is nothing so practical as a good theory" when it comes to conceptualizing the goals and objectives of IPE courses and programs and to developing the research foundation that will be increasingly important to the IPE field itself.

It has also been our attempt to explore and explain some of the key domains of IPE theory, and to indicate why they are such an integral part of teamwork education. Whether there is truly a "unified theory of IPE," or simply differing conceptual foundations for different aspects of it, remains an open question. Regardless, the role of theory in promoting the further development and evolution of IPE as an academic field is assured.

Questions for Discussion

1. Do you use any naive or informal theories in your work in IPE or IPP? By this we mean explanations of things that are happening in either educational or clinical settings that help you to understand them.

2. Do any of the theories presented in this chapter seem particularly relevant to your work in IPE or IPP? How might you use them to improve the effectiveness or efficiency of your interprofessional work?

3. Do you have any other theories you are aware of that might help to expand on the descriptions of theories in this chapter?

11

Developing and Maintaining Interprofessional Education: The Devil Is in the Details[*]

Academia is a highly competitive environment, fraught with vested interests, rigid traditions, and scarce resources. Interdisciplinary education is rarely a primary goal compared to specific knowledge or skill areas, the furtherance of individual disciplines, and the security and advancement of individuals and institutions.

Honesty, trust, and respect are not universal characteristics of higher education, and are subordinate to more pragmatic values, such as survival, security, and advancement. The paucity of resources sharpens the competition between traditional education practices and interdisciplinary education to the disadvantage of the latter.

—David Satin[1]

What has emerged from these experiences with interdisciplinary education and practice is the awareness that the task of teaching cooperation and collaboration in health care is not easy . . . Attempts to promote such

---

[*] Parts of this chapter are based on two previous publications: Clark, P. G. (2011). The devil is in the details: The seven deadly sins of organizing and continuing interprofessional education in the U.S. *Journal of Interprofessional Care*, 25: 321–327; and Clark, P. G. (2013). Towards a transtheoretical model of interprofessional education: Stages, processes, and forces supporting institutional change. *Journal of Interprofessional Care*, 27: 43–49.

efforts seem to meet overwhelming barriers of disciplinary territoriality and systems inertia. As with the mythical Sisyphus, each forward push seems to end with a return to the point of origin, with little tangible evidence of impact or permanence. As a result, each new generation seems to have to repeat the experiences and frustrations of the past.

—DeWitt Baldwin[2]

A Curriculum Development Story

It seems appropriate to start this chapter with a story that is based on the experience of one of us in developing IPE courses and programs in higher education settings. It provides the context for the more general discussion that follows, particularly with regard to the challenges of sustaining IPE once it has been initially established.

Years ago, with grant support from a local foundation, a colleague and I developed a new, interprofessional service-learning course in aging and health at our university. Its focus was on acquiring basic interprofessional teamwork skills and core geriatric competencies for advanced undergraduate and graduate students in the health professions on our campus.

The "seminar" component consisted of weekly classes to discuss assigned readings on teamwork, aging, and health topics. The "service" component involved the students working as a team to develop and deliver six to eight hour-long weekly health promotion workshops for residents at a local housing site for older adults. Faculty from cooperating health professions programs served as mentors for the students in their programs, meeting all together with the students at the beginning and the end of the semester, and individually with each student in their respective programs during the course of the experience.

While there were some initial problems with scheduling to make it possible for students from different programs to participate, the course got off to a strong start. Faculty from the different academic departments were supportive and enthusiastic, readily offering their time and talents to this new venture on an "overload" basis (i.e., not as a part of their regular instructional assignment by their respective departments). Initial evaluations showed positive impacts on student attitudes toward working with older adults and with each other.

The course was approved as an interprofessional option within the academic division in which it was housed (a school including several aging and allied health programs), although there were problems with getting it cross listed in the other participating academic divisions of the university (e.g., nursing, pharmacy, and nutrition). After two years the grant funding ran out, and it was more difficult to continue the course with reduced resources.

Financial pressures mounted on the university and the school within which I was a faculty member to "cover the basic curriculum" and to let go of elective courses that were not considered essential for the core degree requirements or for accreditation and licensure purposes. I continued to teach this course for several years on an "overload" basis; but eventually I became frustrated and angry, and I stopped when it did not get the support and recognition I felt it deserved from the university administration.

After a gap of several years, I reoffered the course on a trial basis, and it was met with a positive, though somewhat guarded, response from key university administrators. With the support afforded by a new federal health professions training grant, I redesigned and reintegrated the course into my normal departmental teaching duties. In addition, I expanded the focus to include populations other than older adults, added problem-based learning (PBL) methods, and was able to get the course listed as a professional elective in some key health programs (e.g., pharmacy).

However, I have not received strong support from the other major academic divisions of the university responsible for training health professions students (e.g., nursing), and practical challenges regarding scheduling and ongoing participation of students from the other programs remain major issues. In spite of support for interprofessional education voiced at the highest levels of the university administration, this endorsement has not trickled down to the level of actually addressing some of the barriers encountered by faculty wishing to do IPE.

The university has recently announced a major effort to reorganize its health professions programs, unifying them within a single academic structure, in an effort to promote more interprofessional education and research. It remains to be seen whether this course will benefit from this new structure, or if it will continue to languish in the backwater of programs that do not fit with identified departmental or disciplinary curricula and degree requirements.

Introduction

This story illustrates some of the fundamental challenges in developing and sustaining IPE in higher educational settings, ones that this chapter will explore and discuss. We have worked in the field of interprofessional education and practice for decades; between the two of us, we have over 70 years of experience in developing, implementing, maintaining, and evaluating IPE and IPP initiatives. This rich historical experience affords us with a unique perspective on the contexts and forces—social, political, and economic—that shape IPE and IPP in the United States.

Questions that come to our minds about the future include the following: Will the development and continuation of interprofessional programs in healthcare settings be similar to, or different from, past history? Have we in the United States now—finally—reached a point where the future stability and continuation of IHTs in a variety of clinical settings will be assured? Or, more likely, will we continue on a rollercoaster of ups and downs for IPE and IPP, with advocacy, support, and funding for them waxing and waning with the shifting sands and shoals of healthcare change in the United States?

How will the growing impact of business and corporate models of health care influence the evolution of IHTs and support for them in constantly changing healthcare systems? In educational settings and institutions, will there be growing governmental and academic support for more interprofessional initiatives in the education of health professions students and professionals? Or, will the traditional resistance of entrenched academic structures and processes mediate against change in support of interprofessionalism in higher education?

Though we have no crystal ball for the future of IPE and IPP, we do have some observations based on the past and an assessment of the current status of efforts to promote interprofessionalism in clinical and educational healthcare settings. We can summarize the past with similar words to the quotations from Satin and Baldwin above—that we have seen ups and downs, growth and retrenchment, and optimism and pessimism over the past 60 or 70 years that efforts have been made to expand the use of IHTs in the United States. Perhaps the current situation may best be described as Dickensian; that is, as "the best of times and the worst of times."

On the positive side, for example, recent influential reports and recommendations from the prestigious Institute of Medicine targeting problems in the U.S. healthcare system[3, 4] have led to highlighting the importance of education for IHTs as a way of addressing them[5] and research for demonstrating their effectiveness.[6] New initiatives by a wide range of health professions' associations have led to the broad-scale endorsement of interprofessional education for IHTs.[7] Special populations, such as older adults, have also been targeted for additional attention to the need for interprofessional care[8, 9] Finally, the advent of new models of primary care based on teamwork in the Patient-Centered Medical Home[10] has further raised the hopes of interprofessional advocates that we have finally turned the corner on the sustainability of IPP.

On other hand, higher educational institutions in the United States—which will need to respond to these initiatives and calls for increased IPP—have traditionally been built around vertical structures or silos, such as departments and schools, that make collaboration across academic units difficult. This is especially the case when resources are in short supply, and the need to "cover the basic curriculum" mediates against efforts that are innovative. Many health professions curricula, such as nursing, are extremely structured, with very few or no electives and little room for the addition of one new idea or initiative. In addition, some health professions, particularly medicine, generally are not supportive of IPE and have a history of not enthusiastically participating in efforts to promote interprofessionalism in the curriculum.

Especially challenging is the continuation or sustainability of interprofessional efforts over the long term. External funding, such as grants, can temporarily lead to the development of new programs; but, as most of us know, when the grant money runs out, institutions usually return to the pre-grant status quo as the academic default setting. Additionally, higher education is typically uncoupled from the clinical sector side, so even if there were demand for interprofessionally trained providers from the healthcare system itself, it would take considerable time and effort for there to be a response from the academic sector. The pipeline between the academic and the clinical setting is very long and twisted, with lots of kinks and variable flows that make a timely and appropriate response uncertain. Finally, it is likely that additional pressures, such as those from licensure and accreditation bodies, will have to be brought to bear before higher education institutions will be responsive to calls for IPE in their curricula.

In light of this uncertain situation and to move our understanding of the complex factors and forces in play to promote IPE, the objective of this chapter is twofold: (1) to provide a comprehensive review of the challenges and barriers to interprofessional efforts in the higher education setting, focusing particularly on the qualities of people and programs that make change difficult, and (2) to develop a framework for designing strategies for change that will move academic institutions in the direction of increased support for interprofessionalism. Throughout this discussion, the emphasis will be on the kinds of approaches, resources, and strategies that can lead to the changes needed if we are to promote the development and continuation of IPE in higher education settings. In addition, we are informed by the history of previous efforts to bring about such changes and guided as much by the failures as the successes of the past.

Challenges to Interprofessional Education

As the quotations at the beginning of this chapter suggest, higher educational institutions are arenas in which personal and professional interests, political power struggles, survival instincts, and resource conflicts are played out on a regular—even daily—basis. Major players in this arena—such as deans—jockey for position, power, and prestige. Higher-level administrators, such as provosts, are often responding to ideological and market forces emanating from the larger academic, social, and economic context. Similarly, faculty are motivated and rewarded to act in certain ways in response to the existing incentive structure within the institution.

An understanding of these factors and forces is necessary before we can even begin to think about how to change them. What follows is an attempt to develop a kind of "personal and political economy of IPE" framework that draws out the power, policies, and politics that are the dominant forces in universities, set against the backdrop of the academic structures of departments and schools. This includes a consideration of: (1) disciplinary dominance, (2) academic arrogance, (3) professional power, (4) IPE lite, (5) resource requirements, and (6) continuous commitment.

Disciplinary Dominance

Disciplines are the core intellectual structures of the university, and they are usually embodied in individual departments or schools. They consist of two major features: (1) the cultural or social, expressed as a community of individuals who collaborate in teaching and research, and (2) the epistemological and linguistic, reflecting shared ways of obtaining, using, and communicating knowledge.[11, 12] They also serve as loci of loyalties and allegiances, and their practitioners (faculty and students) are clustered and cloistered within colleges or schools that make up the larger university. Students are protectively housed within these structures, and faculty members receive incentives for promotion and tenure, as well as power and prestige, for their contributions to them.

Because disciplines provide the major structures and processes of the modern university, attempts to develop crosscutting or interdisciplinary alternatives will always have an uphill struggle to be successful. They always run the risk of being considered peripheral or nonessential; or, even worse, irrelevant and unnecessary.[13] They challenge the predictable order, control, and certainty of disciplinary structures and are a threat to the status quo, vested interests, and established power relationships in an institution.[14] Interdisciplinary programs often exist outside the traditional power structures of the university, with no direct access to resources and decision-making discussions.

For example, at one university with which we are familiar, the chairs of the basic academic units—departments—within the higher-order college unit of the university make up the management team. This group meets on a regular basis with the dean of the college to discuss and shape policies and programs and to review current and future resource allocations within the college and the larger university. The directors of two interprofessional programs within this college are not part of this management group, and are therefore not privy to discussions about issues affecting academic programs and resources. Moreover, they do not directly participate in discussions about new faculty positions or debates about current or future institutional directions. Even worse, the two interprofessional programs are often seen, formally or informally, as simply being a part of the two departments with which they are loosely affiliated.

Because of these factors, interprofessional programs are always under threat from opposing forces that would reverse their development and jeopardize their continuation. Substantial energy must be invested in their preservation, or they will revert to the traditional "default" structures based on disciplines, departments, and deans.

Academic Arrogance

Satin[15] has observed that the "disrespect of subordinate disciplines by superordinate ones" is a major reason for the failure of interprofessional programs. Insofar as different health professions have become differentiated and evolved to become unique, they have had to protect their own status and power, based on ideological, socioeconomic, and political factors.[16, 17] The traditional hierarchical arrangement of the health professions, with medicine at the top, is threatened by a leveling of the playing field dependent on mutual recognition, respect, and reliance on other professions.

For example, evaluations of IPE programs have underscored the reluctance of medicine to participate in them. Reuben and colleagues[18] found that the quality and the extent of medicine's involvement in geriatric IHT programs was less than nursing and social work, on the part of both students and faculty. Physicians are likely to see IPE as a threat to their dominance in clinical settings. This perception is reinforced by the recognition in academic health centers in the United States that medicine is weaker in its support of IPE than nursing and pharmacy, based in part on the belief that such experiences would dilute the essential content needed for medical education.[19] This suggests that IPE, even when present in some health professions programs, is marginalized and seen as an interesting "add on" but not as an activity that is central to the core mission of health professions education.

Professional Power

Power, and the personal and political struggle to attain or retain it, is a key reality in academic settings. In IPE, power is a key component of prestige and status. Insofar as interprofessional programs seek to redistribute power more equally among the participating professions, they will always run the risk of being opposed, actively or passively, by those disciplines in power. Once again, medicine's support for IPE seems problematic. Empirical research suggests that medicine claims more power on IHTs than other professions; for example, medical students believe that physicians, because of their training, should be team leaders, be able to unilaterally change patient care plans developed by a team, and bear ultimate legal responsibility for the patient.[20]

Another evaluation of the same program revealed that medical residents were not interested in IPE participation, because it threatened the biomedical focus of their profession and weakened medicine's power to define the patient's problem.[21] Physicians like to see themselves as leaders and their approach to the patient as the most important, with other professions playing a supportive or secondary role.[22] In the context of academic programs, similar beliefs can undercut or torpedo the development of IPE by overt or covert opposition to its underlying values and objectives.

IPE Lite

Those working in academe are all too familiar with faculty members and administrators who jump on an educational bandwagon that is passing by and seems to offer personal or professional advantages, such as advancement or recognition. There is also the attraction of the intellectual "fad du jour," in which a current "hot topic" or stylish, trendy, or expedient idea attracts academic interest and administrative support. However, educational fads come and go, and the long-term support, commitment, and belief in the core values of IPE may not always be present. IPE may receive superficial support or lip service, but the strong foundation of commitment is lacking. Administrators may "talk the IPE talk," but not "walk the IPE walk" in terms of their contributions of resources over a long time period.

Paradoxically, this temptation toward "IPE lite" is reinforced by the availability of grant funding. Anyone can look interprofessional for a few years if they are getting paid for it by having a training grant. As funding agencies increasingly emphasize interprofessional requirements for successful grant proposals, it is important that they do not unwittingly create a false sense of progress in promoting IPE by supporting academic efforts that are interprofessional in name only. For example, Satin[23] mentions a case in which a prominent medical school set up a "front" IPE program with other health professions schools in the same geographic area just to get a large federal training grant. To no one's surprise, the "floating skyscraper" program evaporated when the funding ended.

Resource Requirements

Adequate resources of different types are essential for the successful development and continuation of IPE in higher education settings. Resources represent a supply of energy to develop a place and a space for IPE, as well as the ability to keep the horizontal collaborative arrangements in place in a setting where vertical structures are the norm. As discussed earlier, grant funding can provide an initial source of this energy, but it is often a double-edged sword if it simply masks the lack of adequate genuine support from administrators that is needed over the long run.

Successful IPE initiatives need more than funding, however. They require other types of academic resources to attract and retain faculty members, such as release time, encouragement and "moral support," and credit at critical times such as promotion and tenure decisions. Moreover, both "bottom up" and "top down" support is essential. Senior administrators need to signal publicly the importance of such programs in meeting high priorities for the institution, and "on the ground" supports such as teaching release time and assistance in addressing logistical barriers to successful program development are equally important.

At their most basic level, resources represent sources of legitimacy and congruence with institutional priorities. If IPE is to succeed and flourish over the long term, it must be hardwired into institutional processes and structures, not simply grafted onto existing disciplinary structures and pruned off when times get tough and resources are more limited. As Barr and Ross[24] suggest from a U.K. perspective, "If 'mainstreaming' is to be more than mere rhetoric, IPE must pervade the culture of professional education, supported unequivocally by top management, backed by the spectrum of stakeholders, benefiting from core educational funding, owned equally by each of the constituent professional programmes, permeating uniprofessional and multiprofessional teaching and learning throughout. Easily said, less easily done!"

Continuous Commitment

Successful continuation of IPE requires long-term commitment from the host institution. Short-term pilot projects, with the expectation of sustainability following a limited duration of support, will not succeed. Administrators must be willing to devote energy and enthusiasm, as well as tangible recognition and resources, over a long period in order to ensure the viability of a new project. Too often in our experience, we have found that administrators have a limited time horizon and unreasonable expectations for success after one or two years of funding.

The other important issue in terms of support is the importance of transcending individual people or personalities. In spite of the essential need for an individual champion to advocate and lobby for an IPE program, long-term success must extend beyond any one person. Faculty and administrators may come and go, but the program must continue. The only way to achieve this outcome is for IPE to be woven into the very fabric of the academic community so that the interprofessional thread is an essential part of the institution. To use a different metaphor, if we truly are to tear down the vertical academic silos constituting the university, and build horizontal bridges between departments and schools, then we must be sure that the bricks we have removed are cemented into their new locations.

Strategies for Promoting and Sustaining IPE

Reviewing the challenges and barriers to IPE should be a sobering reminder of the difficult tasks that lie ahead for anyone who would develop and sustain it over the long term. The "good news" shared at the beginning of this chapter about recent developments in support of IPE give us some hope that positive change is, indeed, possible. To further our thinking about how to bring about the truly systemic change we seek, this section introduces a framework for thinking about change and then some concrete strategies for implementing it.

Frameworks for Change

Organizational change in support of IPE is challenging, but fortunately we have some conceptual tools with concrete applications that can make it easier to develop strategies for its promotion. These include: (1) force field analysis, (2) the transtheoretical model, and (3) higher education change models.

Force Field Analysis

The social psychologist Kurt Lewin[25] developed force field analysis as a framework to think systematically about social or organizational change. It describes any current situation or status quo as being a state of equilibrium between driving forces for change and restraining forces that oppose it. The driving forces are generally positive, reasonable, logical, conscious, and economic; in contrast, the restraining forces are usually negative, emotional, illogical, unconscious, and social–psychological.

The framework suggests that change cannot be achieved only by increasing the forces for change as long as the restraining forces remain in place. Change is easier and more likely to be sustained if the opposing forces are reduced. In addition, there are three stages of change: (1) *unfreezing*, when the strength of forces maintaining the current equilibrium is reduced; (2) *moving*, in which new organizational values, attitudes, and behaviors to help promote change are developed and implemented; and (3) *refreezing*, when the changes that have been made are stabilized to create a new equilibrium.

Transtheoretical Model of Change

Theories of change suggest that a targeted or situation-specific approach to organizational transformation is more effective than a "one size fits all" method, due to the fact that what is needed is a strategy focused on the specific factors related to organizational contexts and the readiness to change of particular individuals or groups within an organization. In addition, comprehensive approaches should suggest different strategies for differing stages of the change process.

One such theory is the transtheoretical model (TTM) of behavior change, originally developed to explain individual behavioral change.[26] Based on an integration of a number of psychosocial concepts and theories, this model suggests that individuals wishing to change go through a series of discrete stages: (1) *precontemplation*, no intention to change in the foreseeable future, (2) *contemplation*, intention to change within the next six months, (3) *preparation*, serious intention to change within the next month, (4) *action*, initiation of change, and (5) *maintenance*, sustaining change for six months or more.

Linked to the stages of change are processes that describe how change occurs. In fact, as the TTM has increasingly been applied to organizations—including higher education institutions—the processes have emerged as particularly crucial.[27, 28] In this context, they describe activities that leaders can employ to facilitate change in a particular direction. Different processes are associated with specific stages of organizational change and may be targeted on individuals, groups, or units at differing points of readiness for change.

The processes and their corresponding stages are:

1. *Precontemplation/Contemplation*: dramatic relief (expressing feelings, such as fear of not, or excitement about, making a change), self-reevaluation (recognizing that change is important for one's values or sense of self), and thinking about commitment.
2. *Preparation*: teams (working with others to prepare for change).
3. *Action*: consciousness-raising (gaining awareness about a problem and its solutions), counterconditioning (substituting alternative behaviors and patterns of thinking), and making a commitment.
4. *Maintenance*: stimulus control (modifying the environment to discourage old behaviors and encourage new ones), helping relationships (using social support for change), and reinforcement management (identifying intrinsic or extrinsic rewards for changing).

Higher Education Change Models

Other institutional change theorists have developed similar frameworks for planned transformation in higher educational settings. For example, Kezar and Lester[29] and Kezar and Elrod[30] have proposed a three-stage model of institutional change with corresponding actions for each:

1. *Mobilization*: In this stage—analogous to the combined precontemplation, contemplation, and preparation stages of the TTM—the system is prepared for change. Preparation includes recognizing the need for change, articulating a vision, mobilizing support, and enlisting leadership. At this point, policies and practices that embody the institutional culture start to be challenged.
2. *Implementation*: At this stage—similar to the TTM action stage—the change is introduced. It includes developing support, generating incentives and rewards, expanding resources, and modifying work responsibilities for the organization's members. Also at this point, new initiatives and supports to maintain the changes start to develop.
3. *Institutionalization*: The system is stabilized in its changed state, as the TTM maintenance stage suggests. This includes incorporating and sustaining changes by integrating them into the organizational value system and culture. A new understanding of what the change represents is reached by the members.

Finally, other academic organizational change researchers[31] emphasize the need for both (1) *intrinsic*, voluntary forces, and (2) *extrinsic*, forced mechanisms to promote organizational change. In this view, three types of pressures lead to organizational change: (1) *coercive forces*, such as pressures from regulatory agencies; (2) *mimetic forces*, stemming from pressures to imitate peer organizations; and (3) *normative forces*, based on professionalization in which values, codes, and standards are imposed by professional licensure and certification and by accreditation agencies.[32]

Summarizing all these frameworks, what is needed to move IPE efforts forward in higher education institutions is an approach to organizational change that both recognizes that change occurs in stages and that tailors individual strategies for change based on where various individuals, groups, and academic units are in terms of their context and readiness for change. The discussion that follows—organized around the three general stages of mobilization, implementation, and institutionalization—highlights the critical factors and forces that promote and sustain change at each level. We will emphasize leadership implications, due to their importance as an organizational characteristic and a facilitator of change.

Implementing Stages and Strategies for Change

Mobilizing for Change: Getting Organized

This stage of readiness for change corresponds with the "unfreezing" step of force field analysis, and it incorporates the following key behaviors: recognizing the need for change, promoting understanding of it, acknowledging that change can be positive and important, galvanizing support and mobilizing leadership, and making a commitment to it. Here there are two important forces at work: academic structures (restraining) and the role of the champion (driving).

As discussed earlier, traditional academic structures, such as departments based on disciplines, constitute forces that resist change. They represent comfortable educational homes for their faculty and student members. This closed community has its own traditions, social organization, reward system, professional status, and language. All these factors create a known environment that is safer than the uncharted waters and threatening territory of interprofessional programs. Addressing this formidable barrier requires that the academic institution be open and flexible in its structure and processes, develop places—such as interprofessional centers or programs—that enable faculty and students to cut across disciplinary boundaries, and find ways to recognize and reward faculty who dare to venture into this intellectual terra incognita.

A key factor driving change is the champion, who is a visionary and cheerleader for change and the problem solver and troubleshooter when difficulties develop. In particular at this stage of change, the champion has a key leadership role in framing the mission of the IPE program and enlisting others in its achievement. With high intrinsic motivation, this individual builds social capital through developing a relationship network to expand the motivational base for change and address opposition when it arises. The potential "down side" of the champion is that the loss of such an individual can jeopardize an IPE program; the solution to this problem is to cultivate the growth and development of a "circle of champions" to expand partnership capital and build the movement.

Implementing Change: Moving into Action

This phase, closely linked to the "moving" phase of Lewin, involves creating new structures, policies, and processes that support reform. Particularly important at this stage of change are mutual trust, altruistic leadership, and the development of organizational structures that promote change. All of these factors may be considered as driving forces, though their existence may also serve to weaken or neutralize restraining forces.

Trust is the linchpin of relationships and partnerships and an important component of the development of social capital—an essential ingredient in promoting IPE. Trust is a key factor in building academic or learning partnerships, and the lack of it is one of the primary reasons that many interprofessional programs fail.[33] If participants do not feel that they are respected and considered as equals, they will not feel secure in their collaborative efforts.

Trust and respect are also both essential ingredients in developing partnership capital, made up of the interrelationships among individuals and their social networks. Social capital is a resource that can sustain collaboration during the ups and downs of external funding and changing academic administrations. Importantly, it is also the basis for distributed leadership, in which the roles and responsibilities of the collaborative are shared among its members.[34]

The importance of organizational support has already been discussed in the previous section of this chapter. Here we wish simply to reiterate the crucial ingredient of intrinsic rather than extrinsic support. The latter include requirements, mandates, pressures, and incentives (such as grants) imposed by others. However, the former is based on self-driven shared interests and mutual goals. The long-term sustainability of an IPE program is based more on the genuine personal and professional commitment of administrators and other leaders than on the allure of the most recent trend in higher education or large sums of grant support. In addition, and as previously stated, successful IPE requires multiple layers of genuine support, from the top administration down to the people "on the ground" in actual program implementation and logistics.

Institutionalizing Change: Forces for Maintaining It

Refreezing in the Lewinian model of change requires its own tailored strategies for success. Sustaining change requires incorporating it into the institutional culture, value system, and norms; it may also be based on a balance between internal and external forces. This is typically the most difficult stage of IPE to maintain. Some institutional theorists suggest that it requires a balance between normative and coercive forces and a reliance on both intrinsic, voluntary, approaches to change and more extrinsic, forced, mechanisms working together.[35, 36] Taken together, maintenance requires a constant infusion of effort and energy to enable programs to exist in an academic environment where the default setting is always a return to the old disciplinary structures and processes.

Internal forces include ongoing organizational vigilance, energy, and support for IPE over the long term as forms of institutional investment. Required are critical investments in faculty support, development, and rewards. Resources must be committed, institutional priorities shaped, and the importance of the interprofessional vision kept in sharp focus. Achieving this goal over the long term requires reorienting and restructuring both faculty and administrators' interests and skills, and beliefs and ambitions.

Particularly germane to this state of sustainability is the development of performance metrics and accountability structures. Measures to track and evaluate the processes and outcomes of IPE should be put into place, reflecting current trends in higher education toward educational outcome assessment. This goal is consistent with recent reports calling for more research on IPE and IPP as a key to their future in both educational and clinical settings.[37]

External forces from governmental departments and professional associations can bring about and stabilize the kinds of changes needed in academic programs to produce healthcare professionals with the skills necessary to practice in IHTs. Higher education institutions are slow in changing to meet external demands for workforce development. If the knowledge or skill to be developed is not evaluated as part of a professional licensure or certification requirement, or required as part of an accreditation standard for the academic program, then it is unlikely that the curriculum will change to include it.

Though these pressures are beginning to be exerted on universities in the United States, it remains to be seen whether they will produce the desired change in support of IPE. Recent reports on IPE have highlighted the need to bring education and practice settings closer together to ensure that healthcare professionals are being given the necessary knowledge and skills in their education to meet the practice demands of the workplace.[38] The emergence of the business model for both health care and higher education has some major implications for thinking about connecting the education and practice settings.

Implications of the Business Model of Education

Over the past two decades, higher education in the United States has increasingly been seen as any other industry, in very much the same way that health care is now seen as a business. Students are considered to be customers who come to the university for the credentials or skill set needed for a job. This is particularly the case in the health professions, where licensure or certification requires appropriate education from an accredited educational program. This commodification of higher education has increasingly been operationalized in the marketing of educational programs and in a focus on return on investment and other "bottom line" indicators of success. Increasingly, the choice of which academic programs to develop or in which to invest is driven by profit-making motives that have, until recently, been seen as inappropriate or, worse, toxic to the educational arena, where ideas and the pursuit of knowledge for its own sake have long been seen as the primary driving force.

For the future of IPE, the question is now whether market forces will provide the demand for, and support the development of, training programs for IHTs. If so, these factors would be external to the educational institution and originate in practice or clinical settings. However, the forces from this sector would themselves likely be based on the business model of health care, which in the past has not shown much support for the development of teamwork. We have experienced settings in which IHTs have been reduced or even eliminated in the pursuit of increased profits through more billable hours of providing care. In addition, healthcare administrators often hire less-well-trained provider staff, such as a person with a bachelor's or even an associate's degree instead of a master's, to save money on salaries. Little or no consideration is given to the fact that the kind of care provided to patients and the ability to participate effectively in an IHT are jeopardized by this staffing decision.

Insofar as the language of business and management may be applied to IHTs, we suspect that the justification for their development will be described in terms related more to organizational efficiency and cost savings than to the more traditional factors in health care involving patient outcomes or quality of life. This situation threatens to undermine the firm foundation needed for highly trained and skilled team members that is represented by their educational preparation and training.

Summary

Ultimately, the achievement of long-term stability for IPE within a higher education setting structured around disciplines and departments will require an accommodation between interprofessionality as a "discourse of innovation" and disciplinarity as the "foundation of tradition" for the university. Rather than being forced to choose between disciplinary and interprofessional discourse, the reality in the long term is that we need both. As "epistemological structures," disciplines provide the fundamental homes within which particular methods of academic work may grow; at the same time, however, we also need the interfaces between these structures to stimulate intellectual synergy and innovation. This dualistic goal can be sustained in a way that provides both highly qualified healthcare professionals and IHT members who can work together to improve patient care and outcomes.

This chapter has surveyed the many barriers and challenges to developing, implementing, and sustaining IPE in the higher educational setting. By doing so, however, we have not intended to suggest that it cannot be achieved or maintained over the long term. Indeed, there are clearly methods that can be strategically employed to move achieving the goal of IPE forward, even in the face of forces that are arrayed against it. The main message of this chapter has been the importance of being mindful of the resources and requirements for the success of interprofessionalism that must be marshaled and utilized in a thoughtful and targeted fashion. As Satin[39] suggests, "Despite its logical advantages and productivity, interdisciplinary education is a hard road to travel, with few guides and only sketchy maps. It requires flexibility, creativity, persistence, and, above all, commitment to find ways of continuing to exist. It can be done."

Questions for Discussion

1. What are some challenges that you personally have encountered in your own institution or setting in developing or sustaining IPE or IPP programs? In your experience, what were the reasons for these problems, and what did you do to try to solve them?

2. Are there any strategies or approaches described in this chapter that you think might have been helpful in addressing these challenges? Why do you think that they would have been effective?

3. Are there any other strategies that you have found to be effective in addressing the resistance to, or reluctance for, change in either academic or practice settings? Why do you think that these approaches have been effective?

4. In the future, what do you think will be the most effective methods or strategies for making sure that IPE and IPP programs survive and flourish beyond their developmental phase?

12

Final Thoughts and Reflections

The obstacle is the path.

—*Zen proverb*

Introduction

Both IPE and IPP are challenging and difficult, more so than most educators and practitioners realize. What makes them so is that they always seem to be on the fringes of educational and healthcare institutions. Whether they will become integrated into the systems in which they are housed will depend on the advocacy and commitment of educators and providers alike, as well as the administrators in both settings. We believe that such conditions can be created, but IPE and IPP are always dependent on the energy and enthusiasm of those who believe that teamwork is important to improving care and its outcomes. Teamwork will not just happen on its own; it requires sustained energy devoted to its development and continuation.

We hope that this book has provided a strong foundation for those in both academia and clinical settings to become more aware of what goes into effective IHTs and the preparation of professionals to work in them. In this respect, the Zen proverb that "the obstacle is the path" reveals that the way forward in promoting both IPE and IPP is to embrace the challenges that lie in the way and to recognize that the path to promoting them requires taking them head on as the requirements for moving forward. Ignoring them and seeking an "alternative route" to our goal will only lead to wrong turns and dead ends.

As we have said earlier in this book, the way toward interprofession-alism has few maps and only sketchy directions. There is no GPS for this location. We can, however, learn from those who have come before us—not only to see what direction they have taken, but also to learn from what worked and, perhaps more importantly, what did not. IPE and IPP are an ongoing journey, and we need to embrace it for what it is. For those of us who have worked for many years in this field, it sometimes feels that we are trapped in a Sisyphean setting where we move forward at great energy and expense, only to slip back and return to where we started and then have to start all over again. The past history of IPE and IPP efforts is littered with efforts and experiences that started out well but did not stand the test of time.

Perhaps this experiential history will give us new insights into where we actually were at those times and what now needs to be done to move forward. Can we really learn from the past, or are its lessons only answers to questions that no one asks anymore? When we recently submitted an abstract to a major international conference on IPE and IPP for a sym-posium that focused on the question of what we can learn from previous projects and programs on IHTs—with a panel consisting of major figures who have worked for many years in this field—we were notified that our submission was not accepted. It is the premise of this book that attention to, and appreciation of, the past as a source of perspective on the present and ideas for the future are critical if we are to avoid making the same mistakes over and over again.

This final chapter is both a compilation and a distillation of the major points, perspectives, and positions of our book. It is at once a summary and a set of recommendations for future strategies for promoting IPE and IPP. What are the crosscutting themes that are woven into a text that surveys a wide range of interprofessional issues? What do we want people who have read this book to remember and take away from it? We include the following topics: (1) the importance of micro and macro contexts, (2) change is the only constant, (3) linking IPE and IPP more effectively, (4) theories, concepts, and models, and (5) the power of people.

The Importance of Micro and Macro Contexts

IHTs do not exist in a clinical vacuum; neither do educational pro-grams to prepare professionals to work in IHTs. Too often, both educators and clinicians fail to recognize that "context matters." There are two levels of context that deserve our attention: micro and macro.

For example, in the micro practice context, IHTs need to be aware of the importance of factors in their own care organization that either promote or inhibit teamwork, as well as the persons and personalities involved in the administration of programs. Teamwork is fragile and vulnerable in all healthcare settings, so it is important that an IHT have good communication with key administrators about its successes and needs. One of those needs is a responsive electronic medical record that supports a team-defined global goal for each patient. The team must be able to effortlessly alter the goal as the patient's care progresses, and the goal must be prominently displayed to core and extended team members as they intervene on behalf of the patient.

IHTs need to be politically and strategically savvy, or at least have members who can play the role of ambassador to key administrators and be advocates for their work within the organization. IHTs must scan the horizon constantly for threats and be proactive in identifying and addressing them. Teams often seem to forget how contingent their existence is and how dependent they are on informed and supportive administrators.

Similarly, at the macro level, we have sketched out the rapidly expanding business model for health care in the United States and the rise of economic and efficiency values as the measure of healthcare outcomes. The ascendancy of profit-based decision making about how resources will be invested in healthcare services promises to have far-reaching impacts on how health care is conceptualized and delivered in the United States. IHTs are affected by these large-scale forces, which threaten the time and other resources needed for effective team functioning. In addition, these economic values impact teams with respect to the training of their members, with the substitution of less-well-educated and less-expensive providers for those who have more education, are paid more, and have more and better skills for addressing complexity. This directly affects the quality of teamwork and the ability of IHTs to provide good care to difficult and complex patients.

Just as clinical teams operate within a specific organizational context—whether a hospital, long-term care facility, or community care agency—so too do interprofessional educational programs operate within a specific academic context, the university in which they are housed. Just as each clinical setting is different, so too is each academic setting unique in terms of the persons and personalities involved. Do key administrators, such as deans and provosts, really support IPE efforts through the provision of tangible resources, or are they more apt to simply give lip service to the requirements for assistance? Are "bottom up" supports readily available for faculty who venture into the often risky and sometimes dangerous uncharted territory of IPE, or are they "on their own" when it comes to instructional assignments, release time, and the all-important promotion and tenure process? Every IPE program needs a champion who serves as the program advocate, cheerleader, and troubleshooter.

Similarly, at the larger-scale national or macro level, higher education is swept by fads, fancies, and financial forces that promise to direct the entire academic enterprise into new and sometimes controversial directions. Mirroring the rise of the business model in health care, the ascendency of the corporate university that views students as consumers and makes decisions about programs based on profit motives and return on investments is increasingly the academy of the present and likely to be that of the future. How such a provider of educational products and services will respond to the need for healthcare professionals trained in teamwork is unclear, but it is certain that market forces will be the predominant influence on academic decision making. The university increasingly sees its role as providing trained workers for jobs, work defined by the market conditions in the world of health care.

Change Is the Only Constant

As we noted in the Introduction to this book, health care has changed dramatically since we wrote the first edition in 2000, and it promises to keep changing in the future in ways we may not even be aware of currently. IHTs are a part of the shifting sands and shoals of health care, and they are influenced by the constantly changing forces that impact on the present and future of healthcare institutions and services. Indeed, they may be even more vulnerable than other forms of healthcare provision, as they always are at risk of being reduced or eliminated due to their marginalized status.

What change means is that advocates and supporters of IHTs and educational programs training professionals to practice in them must be constantly adapting by responding to current trends and anticipating future possibilities. Clinicians and educators are not usually trained to be strategic thinkers who are always assessing driving and restraining forces, as suggested by the Lewinian model of change. However, it is only by observing and responding to changes in the micro and macro contexts that IHTs can be assured of survival by constantly adapting to their changing circumstances. As in nature, if you can't adapt to the changing environment and evolve to meet its demands, you may become extinct. The IHTs of today may become the healthcare dinosaurs of tomorrow.

For example, the increasing use of communication technology in healthcare settings will have profound impacts on the use and sharing of a wide variety of information. The electronic medical record (EMR) can both support and inhibit IHTs, depending on how it is used in the present and further developed in the future. Though the EMR has often been portrayed as key to improved communication among healthcare providers, it is not necessarily a panacea for all the communication woes of the healthcare system. The simple sharing of larger amounts of information among a group of professionals does not guarantee better communication if the members of the IHT do not read it and then process, integrate, and review it as a team.

In addition, it is very easy for the patient "voice" to be lost in a sea of data. Much like the IHT example given in Chapter 1, collecting large amounts of information from each professional on the team does not mean that that information will be processed accurately in a way that focuses on what the patient and the family need or want. The creation of "virtual teams" connected only by electronic communication systems or devices may not improve patient care if the purpose for which the information is collected and shared is lost in transmission and translation. Our experience with providers suggests that often the professional is more interested in entering the information from the medical encounter into the laptop for the EMR than truly interacting with the patient and listening to what he or she is saying. To use Schön's previously discussed metaphor of the reflective practitioner, the scientific information may now be more readily available in the EMR, but the artistic aspect of practice in which the more subtle and value-laden components are found will be weakened. IHTs may find themselves in situations in which they need to advocate for the time and resources to meet face-to-face and in-person when dealing with complex patients with challenging problems.

Similarly, in higher educational settings, interprofessional programs need to constantly be checking the direction and strength of the winds of academic change, interpreting their implications for the development and continuation of programs that are on the margins of most universities. However, this does not mean they should pursue every intellectual or professional fad that comes along, just to be riding the current academic wave. Indeed, some trends, such as the corporatization of the university, may need to be opposed or at least tempered. Others, such as the use of academic standards that support IPE, may need to be advocated for or strengthened. This may mean working at the national level with organizations that have responsibility for the accreditation of health professions programs. Currently in the United States, national professional organizations and centers dedicated to the promotion of IPE and IPP are working on these kinds of initiatives, trying to exert what leverage they can to support an expansion of IHTs.

Linking IPE and IPP More Effectively

This book has dealt with both IPE and IPP to make an important point: They have to be linked and the connections made stronger and more evident. As increased attention is devoted to global health issues and matching the healthcare workforce to the needs of the future,[1] advocates for IHTs must work to forge stronger links between clinical and community care settings and the higher education institutions that supply their workforce. Traditionally, academic institutions have been distantly removed from the realities of the practice setting, at least in terms of future forces that are driving the need for certain types of skills in healthcare providers. While academic programs in the health professions may have clinical placement sites, the focus is typically on the narrow practice demands and the knowledge and skills needed for successful completion of the specific program and subsequent licensure and certification. The pipeline from demand in clinical settings to the supply in the academic context is typically long and twisted, with lots of kinks and bottlenecks along the way. Universities are notoriously slow to turn in a different direction and change course, to develop new programs, and to be responsive to emergent trends in the workplace.

Grants from such sources as private foundations and the federal government may be of some assistance, but the projects they support often fall victim to the shortcomings of externally funded programs outlined in the previous chapter. If IPE and IPP are to be more closely joined, they will require more systematic and systemic change to unfreeze, move, and refreeze structures and processes. In this case, it is easier to effect change if the forces against change are reduced in strength. For example, efforts currently under way to provide financial incentives to care provider organizations to reduce hospital readmission rates typically associated with difficult and challenging patients may open an opportunity for IHTs to better manage such patients. The Patient-Centered Medical Home may also provide a hospitable location for enhanced teamwork, though this will depend on whether truly interprofessional teamwork and adequately trained providers will be supported in this care model.

Of course, the other side of IPE–IPP transformation is to place increased demand on academic institutions to supply the skilled workforce needed to practice on an IHT. Here, providers, provider organizations, and professional associations have an opportunity to exert pressure on universities to develop more teamwork training options. Working with academic programs to support IPE at clinical training sites at which groups of different health professions students are placed would be a start. We are seeing developments of these types of programs now in the United States, and there is guarded optimism that we may finally be turning a corner on interprofessional programs. However, the ultimate test will be to see how sustainable the outcome is. Shortening the IHT pipeline between education and practice will require the determination and resolution of a wide array of stakeholder groups and organizations to make sure that a longer pipeline with too many branches and dead ends does not grow back.

Theories, Concepts, and Models

Our book has also emphasized the importance of developing and using theories, concepts, and models in both IPE and IPP. Much of IHT practice is based on the erroneous assumption that teamwork is easy, anyone can do it, and it does not require the development of an extensive knowledge and skills base. In fact, the real problem is that practitioners and educators do not know what they don't know. This book is an effort to correct this misperception and to provide the tools needed to develop a systematic understanding of IPE and IPP. Such an understanding is critical in avoiding the phenomenon of floating skyscrapers in both clinical and educational settings. These are structures that seem impressive, but in reality they have no foundations on the solid ground of good theory or conceptual adequacy.

We have taken a lot of time to develop frameworks that organize key aspects and components of topics such as communication, conflict, and leadership. Many chapters have figures and tables that present this information in manageable and usable forms that illustrate interrelationships among different aspects of the same topic. We have, where possible, used research-based information that systematically develops each chapter's focus to show the interrelationships among the different components, along with examples and stories to illustrate important dimensions and aspects. Overall, the emphasis has been on connecting practice knowledge and skills to the underlying theories and concepts that explain why things are important and how they can be understood.

Over the years, we have taught many courses and offered numerous workshops on IHTs, and a common response from participants has often been that "we didn't realize that there is so much information on teamwork!" This is true in both educational and clinical settings, though the theories and concepts are not always relevant to each other and to both contexts. Part of our effort in these courses and workshops has been to offer frameworks and structures with which to organize the information and skills presented or used. The ability to see interrelationships among key factors is an essential element in practicing and teaching teamwork. It's also a part of developing more skilled practitioners for IHTs and educators who can prepare them for IPP.

IPE and IPP are maturing as a distinct field with two faces: one educational and one clinical. The field is beginning to experience the development and expansion of a theoretical base, as is the case for any evolving and growing discipline as it matures and develops a distinct identity. Hopefully, this evolution will continue, and we will see the development of actual academic programs in IPE and IPP, with graduate degrees offered and more research into the impacts of interprofessionalism. The recent Institute of Medicine report[2] on the need for research into the outcomes of IHTs in clinical practice and their effects on patient care is a good example of this development. We are also beginning to see the formation of communities of practice around the development of more theoretical bases and conceptual sophistication in IPE and IPP—frameworks that can be used when developing educational programs, research projects, and clinical settings involving IHTs.

We hope that the readers of this book have developed sufficient insight into, and acquired a level of comfort with, theories, concepts, and models that they can begin to use in their educational and practice settings. Indeed, there is "nothing so practical as a good theory," and this is nowhere truer than in IPE and IPP. We have recently been involved in workshops at international meetings that have focused on promoting the expanded use of theory in both educational and practice settings, and we sense that there is growing interest in, and excitement about, the potential application of theory in addressing concrete challenges in curriculum development, research, and clinical care.

The Power of People

Finally, the advancement and sustainability of IPE and IPP depend on individuals and groups of people who are committed to them over the long haul. If there is anything that the history of efforts in this area reveals, it is the critical need for champions to play the role of advocates at the local and national levels. The progress that has been made in the past is directly tied to persons and professionals who were committed to IHTs and were willing to devote their careers to developing and supporting the continuation of healthcare teamwork. This lineage of supporters and advocates must be extended if we are to see IPE and IPP move forward, prosper, and be sustained into the future.

At the clinical or practice level, this might include healthcare professionals with teamwork training playing the role of IHT coordinator. Here, it is important to remember that leadership on IHTs can take many forms, but one of the most important is the role of organizer or advocate. Often at the end of courses or workshops we have offered, we will make it clear to participants that they now should be empowered to assume responsibility for supporting IHTs within their practice or educational institutions. One of us even went to the length once of handing out toy "sheriff's badges" at the end of a workshop, illustrating how participants were now "deputized" to be IHT advocates and champions, once they returned to their healthcare work setting. While this may sound a bit corny, the reality was that participants got the point about how their new-found IHT knowledge invested them with the responsibility to use it as team leaders.

Similarly, in the educational context, faculty advocates for the development and continued support of IPE need to be encouraged and rewarded for their efforts and endeavors, which may, in some contexts, put their academic advancement up the disciplinary ladder in some jeopardy. Insofar as some academic institutions are now creating interprofessional programs in the health disciplines, it is important that the faculty—particularly junior faculty—receive the top-down and bottom-up support that the literature indicates is needed for the successful development, implementation, and continuation of IPE. We are starting to see some academic institutions actually recruiting new faculty who have interprofessional experience in certain areas, such as gerontology, where it is an important contribution to the field of study. While this is certainly a positive development, it is one that needs to be encouraged in the future to continue and grow.

Finally, in both educational and practice contexts, the role of administrative leadership is critical for interprofessional programs to take root and flourish. The need for support—both tangible in terms of concrete resources and intangible in terms of moral and intellectual contributions—is a critical factor in the success of both IPE and IPP. In fact, we really need to consider administrators a member of the team, due to their critical leadership role in making it possible for IHTs to exist and survive during times of change in the healthcare system. Of course, this also means that IHT members and academic program faculty need to keep administrators informed about their important contributions to such key outcomes as student success and patient care improvement. Also, since administrators come and go, it is essential that such education and information be provided on an ongoing and continuing basis.

Final Observations

If you have stayed with this book and read all the chapters to this ending, you are to be congratulated! You now know considerably more about IHTs and the conditions needed for their success. We have appreciated your letting us share several decades of experience with IHTs with you. It is our hope that at least some readers of this book will go on to become the new leaders in the next generation of advocates and champions for IPE and IPP. Although we have often found this road to be a challenging and at times frustrating and discouraging one, we are glad that we embraced the Zen proverb that "the obstacle is the path" and claimed this road as ours over decades of interprofessional work. For us, it has been a rewarding journey, as we hope it will also be for you.

Questions for Discussion

1. What is the most important or personally relevant insight or idea that you can take away from this book? Why is it important for you, and how do you intend to use it?
2. What are some concrete steps that you can take in your institution or organization to become a stronger advocate or champion for IPE and IPP?

Appendix 1: Resources for Interprofessional Practice and Education

The following list of national and international associations and organizations, resource centers, position statements, curricula, journals, and team development measures represents resources that may be helpful in your interprofessional practice and education activities.

National and International Associations and Organizations

American Interprofessional Health Collaborative
http://www.aihc-us.org

Canadian Interprofessional Health Collaborative
http://www.cihc.ca

European Interprofessional Practice and Education Network
http://www.eipen.eu

Nordic Interprofessional Education Network
http://nipnet.org

Australasian Interprofessional Practice and Education Network
http://www.aippen.net

Japan Interprofessional Working and Education Network
http://jipwen.dept.showa.gunma-u.ac.jp

The (U.K.) Centre for the Advancement of Interprofessional Education
  http://caipe.org.uk

All Together Better Health
  http://www.atbh.org

Resource Centers

National Center for Interprofessional Practice and Education
  https://nexusipe.org

Position Statements on IPE and IPP from National and International Organizations

Institute of Medicine

Interprofessional Education for Collaboration: Learning How to Improve Health from Interprofessional Models across the Continuum of Education to Practice (2013)
  http://iom.nationalacademies.org/Reports/2013/Interprofessional
  -Education-for-Collaboration.aspx

Josiah Macy Foundation

Educating Nurses and Physicians: Toward New Horizons: Advancing Interprofessional Education in Academic Health Centers (2010)
  http://macyfoundation.org/docs/macy_pubs/JMF_Carnegie_Summary
  WebVersion%283%29.pdf

Team-Based Competencies: Building a Shared Foundation for Education and Clinical Practice (2011)
  http://macyfoundation.org/docs/macy_pubs/Team-Based
  _Competencies.pdf

Conference on Interprofessional Education (2012)
  http://macyfoundation.org/docs/macy_pubs/JMF_IPE_book
  _web.pdf

Transforming Patient Care: Aligning Interprofessional Education with Clinical Practice Redesign (2013)
  http://macyfoundation.org/docs/macy_pubs/JMF_Transforming
  PatientCare_Jan2013Conference_fin_Web.pdf

Interprofessional Care Coordination: Looking to the Future (2013)
  http://macyfoundation.org/docs/grantee_pubs/NYAM_Issue_Brief
  -Care_Coordination.pdf

*Partnering with Patients, Families, and Communities to Link Interprofes-
  sional Practice and Education* (2014)
  http://macyfoundation.org/docs/macy_pubs/JMF_PartneringwithPFC.pdf

Partnership for Health in Aging, American Geriatrics Society

*Position Statement on Interdisciplinary Team Training in Geriatrics: An
  Essential Component of Quality Health Care for Older Adults* (2014)
  http://www.americangeriatrics.org/pha/partnership_for_health_in
  _aging/interdisciplinary_team_training_statement

World Health Organization

*Framework for Action on Interprofessional Education and Collaborative
  Practice* (2010)
  http://www.who.int/hrh/resources/framework_action/en

Interprofessional Curricula

Hartford Institute for Geriatric Nursing

Geriatric Interdisciplinary Team Training (GITT)
  http://hartfordign.org/education/gitt

Agency for Healthcare Research and Quality

TeamSTEPPS Primary Care Version
  http://www.ahrq.gov/professionals/education/curriculum-tools
  /teamstepps/index.html

Journals

Journal of Interprofessional Care
  http://www.tandfonline.com/toc/ijic20/current

Journal of Interprofessional Education and Practice
  http://www.journals.elsevier.com/journal-of-interprofessional
  -education-and-practice

Journal of Research in Interprofessional Practice and Education
  http://www.jripe.org/index.php/journal

Team Development Measures

Heinemann, G. D., and Zeiss, A. M. (Eds.). (2002). *Team performance in health care: Assessment and development.* New York: Kluwer Academic/ Plenum Publishers.

Stock, R., Mahoney, E., and Carnety, P. (2013). Measuring team development in clinical care settings. *Family Medicine, 45*: 691–700.

Other

Bumann, M. J., and Younkin, S. (2012). Applying self efficacy theory to increase interpersonal effectiveness in teamwork. *Journal of Invitational Theory and Practice*, 18: 11–18.

Howell, T. (2015). The Wisconsin Star Method: Understanding and addressing complexity in geriatrics. In M. L. Malone, E. Capezuti, and R. M. Palmer (Eds.), *Geriatric models of care: Bringing 'best practice' to an aging America* (pp. 87–94). Switzerland: Springer International Publishing.

Appendix 2: Case Studies and Exercises for Interprofessional Education

The following exercises, case studies, and accompanying discussion questions are provided as training resources for both educational and practice settings. They can be altered and may be used in applying the ideas and concepts from the different chapters in this book.

Case #1: Healthcare Teamwork in a Business-Driven Environment

Developing and Maintaining Teams

Your healthcare facility has decided to transform itself into an interprofessional team environment. They have recently sent 20 teams of three (nurse, nurse practitioner, and physician) to the TeamSTEPPS training program. Administrators have also identified one team member on each team to be the team manager. Some of the social workers, clinical pharmacists, dietitians, and rehabilitation staff who cover several teams feel like second-class citizens. They want the training to include them as well. Some of the team managers would like to conduct team training for all members of the team but many of them are concerned about their own time limits since they are still expected to see patients. Some of the nurse team managers have been complaining about a few physician team members who are acting out. The nurse managers not only do not feel comfortable counseling team members from other disciplines about their maladaptive behaviors, but they feel a few of the physicians who are acting in an arrogant manner might go over their heads and try to get them fired. Several of the nurse managers have contacted administration about these problems but the administrator they spoke with simply said that everyone was a professional and must be reminded to behave in a professional manner. He also said if it wasn't interfering with patient care they should ignore the behaviors. The problems have continued.

Questions for Discussion

1. What elements of teamwork are present and what elements are missing in this case?
2. What is the next step for the team managers?
3. What can be done to strengthen the current teams?
4. What should the roles of administration be in this case?

Case #2: Communication

Fractured Humerus

Friday evening in a small town a woman, age 70, was walking her dog and fell on her shoulder. An on-call physician examined her in the ER. In addition to abrasions, the ball of the woman's humerus was crushed and rotated. The woman was discharged home with a recommendation she take over-the-counter pain medicine and she was scheduled to see the surgeon on Monday. Saturday the woman was in excruciating pain and could not sleep. Sunday afternoon the woman could no longer tolerate the pain and called her regular doctor who offered to admit her to the hospital. Upset, the woman refused admission.

The doctor prescribed a scheduled pain medication but the on-call pharmacist could not be reached and the doctor called the prescription in to another pharmacy 40 miles away. When the woman's husband arrived to pick up the medicine the pharmacist said he could not fill the prescription without a signature from the doctor. The husband refused to leave without the medicine and the pharmacist agreed to fill the prescription knowing that he could be cited for violating the law.

Questions for Discussion

1. How could this patient have received better care?
2. What are the structures and processes of communication that could have helped this patient?

Case #3: The Patient as Teacher and Learner

Mrs. Teresa Medeiros

Introduction

You are a member of an assessment IHT working at Central Hospital in the city. Your team routinely gets referrals from inpatient units and the emergency department (ED) at the hospital.

Your core IHT consists of a physician, nurse, pharmacist, and social worker. However, other healthcare professionals can be called in on an "as needed" basis.

Case

Mrs. Teresa Medeiros is an 82-year-old woman who has been referred to your team for assessment. She has been diagnosed with diabetes and congestive heart failure and has been seen at the hospital's ED three times in the past month. She is considered to be a "problem patient" or a "gomer" and has been labeled as "noncompliant" by the ED staff.

Mrs. Medeiros has lived alone for the past 12 years, since her husband died. She resides in a senior housing apartment building in the local community. Fluent in Portuguese, she has limited English-speaking and -reading skills. Before retiring, she worked for many years in a local jewelry manufacturing plant in the city.

Her daughter usually accompanies her mother for doctor's visits, but she has been having health problems of her own and has not been able to help her mother recently.

Questions for Discussion

1. What specific issues would your team be concerned about? Why?
2. What types of assessments would the different members of your IHT perform?
3. What factors do you, as a team, think would be most relevant to Mrs. Medeiros's care?
4. What would your team recommend as interventions to address these factors?
5. What do the different professions on your team each contribute to putting together a complete picture of Mrs. Medeiros's health problems, including, especially, her health literacy?
6. How should Mrs. Medeiros be involved in the team's discussion?

Case #4: Conflict, Patient Involved Care

A female, age 20, was being prepped for eye surgery and the nurses noticed she had a very elevated blood pressure. The nurses had peeled down the patient's gown as they were setting up the leads. Just then a doctor appeared outside the curtain saying that he was coming in. One of the nurses said, "Oh no you don't, we are setting up an EKG and the patient isn't ready to receive you." The physician said, "It is nothing I haven't seen before." The nurse repeated, "You cannot come in yet." Finally the nurses were finished and the physician appeared again saying, "I have seen it all before." The patient was quite embarrassed and simply glared at him, not speaking until the physician apologized for his behavior.

Questions for Discussion

1. How should the team handle this situation after the fact?
2. How should they involve the patient in the discussion?

Case #5: Team Leadership

You are a member of an interprofessional oncology team at a large hospital. Two days ago one of the team's oncology patients died after a long and painful illness. The family obituary stated that his death was "due to doctors." Hospital management is aghast and there is whispering about your team. Negative publicity in the past has led to reduced admissions and resulted in layoffs. The newspaper has called the hospital CEO for an interview for their special report on "Hospital Care Run Amok?" The team medical director wants to know how the team is going to present itself at a meeting scheduled with the hospital CEO.

Questions for Discussion

1. Who should lead the team in addressing this situation?
2. What other types of leadership might be valuable in this situation?

Case #6: Conflict, Values, Ethics

The Resident

A patient fell one evening and was admitted to the hospital with a fractured hip. Diagnoses included end-stage dementia. The medical resident on the geriatric team's service who saw the patient in the ED worked him up and consulted orthopedics for a surgical consult. The next morning the patient was presented in the team meeting and the social worker asked the resident if she had questioned the family about their desire for surgery. The resident became upset and defensive saying the patient had presented to the ED and the standard of care was work-up and surgical intervention for a broken hip. The resident also said that she did not think a social worker should question a physician's medical judgment.

Questions for Discussion

1. What types of conflict are represented in this case?
2. What are your suggestions for resolving the conflicts?

Case #7: Healthcare Teamwork in a Business-Driven Environment

Patient Privacy Officer

A long-term healthcare facility serves clients with chronic care and mental health needs. The clients are in three levels of care: independent living, assisted living, and long-term care. The privacy officer was concerned about compliance with the HIPAA regulations and objected to having the client's names on the doors to their rooms. Some of the nurses and social workers thought this was crazy because it was a way for many of the clients to recognize their rooms. They chose to ignore the admonition of the privacy officer. The privacy officer became more adamant in her ruling and ordered housekeeping to remove the signs saying the nurses and social workers had no business telling administration what to do.

Questions for Discussion

1. What type of conflict is this?
2. What conflict management approaches might be helpful?
3. What elements of teamwork are missing in this situation?
4. What types of team leadership would be most helpful in resolving this conflict?
5. What are some solutions to this conflict?

Case #8: Healthcare Teamwork in a Business-Driven Environment

Developing and Maintaining Teams

I am a supervisor within a large healthcare system with many centers across the state. Each center houses IHTs with clients who have multiple mental and physical problems. Each team consists of several RNs, an NP, home health workers, an administrative assistant, and a social worker. The teams coordinate care with physicians in community clinics. In addition to my supervisory duties I am team manager for five teams. I help the teams identify conflicts and leadership issues and also help them solve frequent problems that arise. The teams generally function very well and benefit from having easy access to my counsel. Recently my boss told me she would like me to assume the job of training teams around the state. She said it was too costly to have team managers devoted to developing and maintaining the teams. She also said the teams were capable of managing themselves.

Questions for Discussion

1. What elements of teamwork are absent from this scenario?
2. At what point is an IHT able to manage itself?
3. What is the purpose of a team manager?

Case #9: Conflict, Ethics, and Patient and Family Involved Care

The Caregiver

Jan is a 62 year old living at home with a diagnosis of cirrhosis of the liver. Her primary caregiver is her 44-year-old son, Barry, who is single and is very emotional about mother's illness and disease process. Barry mentioned to the RN that he didn't know if he could handle the situation if his mother stopped eating. Barry rejected the use of a feeding tube saying, "I am not going to give up and I will keep feeding her as long as I can." Later in the afternoon, Barry stated to the bath aide that he would put a pillow over his mother's face if she could no longer eat or drink. The conversation was reported to the team nurse. The nurse practitioner feels that Adult Protective Services should be contacted. The social worker is concerned but feels that calling in Protective Services will jeopardize the team's ability to work with the family.

Questions for Discussion

As a group:

1. What are the conflict(s), if any?
2. What are the sources or potential sources of the conflicts?
3. What are the type(s) of conflict(s) in this case?
4. What are possible approaches to the conflict(s)?
5. What would your team's approach be to involving the patient's caregiver in the discussion?

Case #10: Ethics

Gertrude Camebo

Mrs. Gertrude Camebo is an 82-year-old divorced female with Type II insulin-dependent diabetes, hypertension, vascular dementia, prior cerebrovascular accident with left-sided weakness, angina, and a history of falls. She has prescriptions for six medications that require a complex dosing regimen. Mrs. Camebo has an income from Social Security and her former husband's pension that puts her above the income limit for support services. She lives in her own home with her only child, a daughter, the daughter's husband, and their teenage son. Mrs. Camebo has told them they can live in her house as long as they help her get by. The daughter works part time as a grocery store bagger and the son-in-law is looking for work. Although the daughter appears fond of her mother, she seems unable to comprehend her mother's disabilities. For example, the daughter expects her mother to do her own laundry, which is in the basement of her home. Mrs. Camebo has fallen numerous times in the past year—once down the basement stairs. She was treated for a concussion and hospitalized briefly for observation after she fell and sustained multiple abrasions.

After her most recent fall, Mrs. Camebo was referred for a competency hearing at which the judge ruled her mentally competent. She reiterated to the social worker that she wanted to live at home. Although the daughter says she understands her mother's medication regimen, medication reviews and blood glucose levels indicate poor compliance. A community-based home healthcare team that provides Mrs. Camebo's care suspects her falls may be due in part to the noncompliance. Also, the house needs extensive repairs, inside and out, and it could use railings on both sides of the stairways. The home health social worker found a repair service that would install the railings at cost. However, the daughter said that they do not have the money. The IHT has evaluated Mrs. Camebo's activities of daily living (ADLs) and also her instrumental activities of daily living (IADLs). She appears to be independent in most of her ADLs. However, she needs help with many of her IADLs, like shopping, cleaning, money management, home repair, medication management, meal preparation, and transportation.

Mrs. Camebo's son-in-law drinks heavily and has difficulty holding a job. He is home alone with her during the day when his wife is at work. All of the falls have occurred when the daughter is at work. The nurse on the team suspects that the son-in-law may be responsible for several falls.

However, the social worker notes that the team has absolutely no proof of any abuse. Although she appears somewhat depressed, Mrs. Camebo's medical conditions are currently stable. Because of this, Medicare guidelines will not support continued home visits.

At the weekly IHT meeting there is considerable discussion about Mrs. Camebo's safety at home and whether there is abuse and/or neglect occurring in the household. The physician favors a more aggressive approach to the situation and recommends reporting the current circumstances to the state authorities for an investigation. She also admits she has been "liberal in documenting disabilities" to permit continued monitoring by home care. The registered nurse on the team, who is a close friend of the agency's administrator, accuses the doctor of Medicare fraud, saying the doctor is being irresponsible in her behavior, and she threatens to report the MD. The social worker is shocked. He feels the nurse is behaving in a heartless manner and tells her he does not think it is a good idea to report anyone. The rest of the team's members (occupational therapy assistant, nursing assistant, and licensed practical nurse) are silent.

Questions for Discussion

1. What are the ethical issues at stake in this case?
2. How do they affect the work of the IHT in deciding what to do in this situation?
3. How should these issues be resolved in a way that is consistent with ethical principles, structures, and processes?

Case #11: Ethics, Team Development, and Conflict

Josephine La Rue

Mrs. Josephine La Rue is a 74-year-old, long-term care facility resident with chronic obstructive lung disease from smoking a pack of cigarettes a day for 60 years. She also has osteoarthritis and mild dementia of unknown etiology, although she has not been judged incompetent. Mrs. La Rue's daughter lives in another city and visits her mother three or four times a year. She says that she often feels guilty that she cannot visit as often as she would like. Mrs. La Rue's daughter has told the social worker that she is visiting long-term care facilities in her area so she can move her mother closer with the hope of visiting her every day. However, the social worker does not feel the daughter is sincere in this desire. The social worker also does not feel a responsibility to help the daughter find another facility as the administrator has informed the staff they need to do everything they can to keep private pay residents happy so they stay at the facility.

Mrs. La Rue had been treated at a local hospital for pneumonia and was returned to the long-term care facility (in which she had spent the past year as a private pay resident) with a prognosis of "probable recovery." The physician who treated her in the hospital was the same physician who cared for her in the facility. However, he had been extremely hard to reach as he was carrying an extra caseload for another physician who was on maternity leave.

Mrs. La Rue's condition started to deteriorate during the two days after readmission to the long-term care facility. She developed a slight fever (99.7 degrees) and she seemed more lethargic. The IHT discussed Mrs. La Rue's case at the weekly team meeting, two days after her discharge from the hospital. The RN, LPN, and social worker on the floor were regular attendees at the weekly meeting. However, the RN who attended this meeting was called to a family emergency during the meeting and was not present for the discussion of Mrs. La Rue's condition. The nursing assistant who was assigned to care for her had mentioned several times to the LPN that, since her return, Mrs. La Rue had expressed a wish to die.

The discussion at the meeting centered on Mrs. La Rue's condition. The RN felt her current status was a remnant of the infection and had planned to inform the physician of significant changes in her condition if the fever increased or if her physical status deteriorated further. The RN said she wanted the staff to closely monitor Mrs. La Rue's vital signs and to alert her if anything changed. After the RN left, the LPN mentioned several times that Mrs. La Rue had expressed her wishes to the staff for no extraordinary measures and that she did not want to be resuscitated. Mrs. La Rue died that night in her sleep.

Mrs. La Rue's daughter informed the state long-term care survey office of her mother's "untimely death." Following an investigation, a state surveyor noted that "the facility did not immediately inform the physician of significant changes in the resident's condition, creating a substantial probability for the resident's death." One staff member, the LPN, who was asked to explain the notification delay, told surveyors that Mrs. La Rue had an advance directive indicating that she did not want to be resuscitated. The facility received a class one violation for this incident and the facility director is furious with the team.

Questions for Discussion

1. What are the issues in this case related to how the IHT is functioning, and how do they affect the work of the IHT and the untimely death of Mrs. LaRue?

2. How should the IHT proceed to address the current situation?

3. What should the role of administration be in relation to the team?

4. How should these issues be resolved in a way that is consistent with ethical principles, structures, and processes?

Case #12: Ethics, Conflict, and Team Decision Making

Happy Sleeper Health Care Center

You are a health professional who is a member of the admissions committee at the Happy Sleeper Healthcare Center. Happy Sleeper is the only long-term healthcare facility within a 200-mile radius and staffing is limited. A group home is the only other long-term care service in the community. Despite this, Happy Sleeper is a well-run facility with concerned staff. Openings only occur about every six months. The admissions committee recently received five applications, postmarked with the same date. The committee is meeting this afternoon to determine which two of the five applicants will be admitted. The applicants are as follows:

Biographical Information

Applicant 1. Roberta: White, Female, Age 89

Roberta is a widow who is a retired farm wife with many infirmities of age. She is hard of hearing, has early dementia, and gets agitated by unfamiliar routines. She also has Parkinson's disease and has had increased difficulty rising and sitting and performing some of her activities of daily living. During her last hospitalization she was diagnosed with MRSA. She has been lovingly cared for by her daughter for 10 years. Her daughter has developed multiple sclerosis and can no longer care for her. Roberta's son, who abuses alcohol, said he would take her in if he had to. Recently Roberta's grandson described her as "the meanest old woman in the world."

Applicant 2. Dewey: Black, Male, Age 67

Dewey, a retired schoolteacher, is a recent widower with severe congestive heart failure. He has had a left hemisphere stroke and has right-sided paralysis. He frequently aspirates when he eats and is malnourished. Dewey has difficulty with verbal communication and becomes very frustrated at times. He served some time for sexually abusing his granddaughter but he was paroled for health reasons. He denies the abuse. He also has a history of having abused his wife and exhibits frustration by striking out with his cane. He has no close family.

Applicant 3. Lyla: White, Female, Age 80

Lyla, a recent widow, is a retired journalist who was known as a "party girl" in her youth. She has severe congestive heart failure, hypertension, and osteoarthritis in her spine. She walks 15–20 feet with a three-wheeled walker. She lives with her daughter who hires someone to stay with her mother while she works. Her daughter says she can no longer provide the help Lyla needs. Lyla is HIV positive from an affair that she had while still married. Lyla is appreciative of any help that is given to her but has been more irritable lately and has been playing her daughter against the woman who comes to stay with her. Lyla has been going downhill since her husband died and is unable to see clearly enough to administer her medicine. She has no other relatives and the local group home has refused to accept her.

Applicant 4. Sam: Hispanic, Male, Age 65

Sam is a retired janitor who has been divorced five times. He has had below the knee amputations of both legs as a result of severe peripheral vascular disease brought on by smoking three packs of cigarettes per day for 50 years. Sam believes someone is out to get him and is constantly calling his congressional representative to complain about the medical establishment. After abusing alcohol for many years, Sam stopped drinking two years ago. Sam is losing weight and says he has trouble chewing. He has recently been diagnosed with stage-3 colon cancer. Although he has three children, each one claims to be too poor to take him in.

Applicant 5. Billybob (as his friends call him): White, Male, Age 55

Billybob, a former owner of an oil-drilling company, lost his business and his fortune through heavy gambling. He was accused and acquitted (on a technicality) of killing his wife 30 years ago. Billybob has COPD with continuous oxygen, is an insulin-dependent diabetic, and has manic-depressive episodes and early dementia. He has had a right hemisphere stroke with weakness in his left leg and falls frequently. Lately, Billybob has been complaining of jaw pain on his left side but the staff thinks it is his way of getting attention. While in the hospital, Billybob was found in the in-service room fondling Resusci-Annie. He has been pinching the female residents in the group home and they want him out. His third wife says she cannot care for him and does not want him back home.

Note to Instructor: This exercise works with multiple small groups. Give each group member five minutes to individually decide on two applicants. Give the groups about 20 minutes to reach a group decision and compare the group decision to the individual decisions within the group. Among the members of the large group, discuss and compare reasons for differences between the choices made by the small groups.

Questions for Discussion

1. What criteria did each group member use to choose two candidates for admission?
2. What criteria did each of the small groups use?
3. What methods of conflict resolution did your group use to resolve conflicts between group members? Were the conflict methods you chose effective? Did they lead to outcomes that were acceptable for your group?

Case #13: Differing Values, Conflict, Ethics, Leadership

The Case of Dr. James

I am a psychologist who is a team member in an outpatient geriatric assessment team that is part of an academic teaching hospital and its healthcare system. Dr. James, a geriatrician, is director of the assessment program. He is a prominent physician within this system and is well liked and respected by his peers. One thing that really bothers me is when he refuses to reveal the diagnosis of dementia to patients and their close family members because "they aren't ready to receive the information." This attitude is problematic when the patient is still driving and during my interviews with the patient's spouse I discover the patient's driving and other behaviors have become risky to the patient and others.

Over time I came to realize that the situation was much more complicated. Because Dr. James likes being "adored" by his patients and he does not like giving them bad news. Another issue was that Dr. James is on the board of this proprietary hospital and they are very concerned about their position within the very competitive communitywide healthcare arena. They do not want to lose patients. In a conversation I had with Dr. James, he admitted that he was concerned about the clinic's ability to attract more referrals and he reminded me our mission was "to provide hope to patients and their families." While Dr. James's behavior violates my code of ethics, the other team members either do not seem concerned or just choose to ignore his behavior. I am torn between organizing the other team members to take a stand or to simply move on to another job.

Questions for Discussion

1. What are the differing values in this situation?
2. What is the best approach to addressing the conflict in values?
3. What ethical dilemmas does this situation present?
4. What kinds of leadership opportunities does this situation present?
5. If you were a team member on this team, what would you do about addressing these issues?
6. How could the team work together to address this situation and who would the team involve?

Case #14: Communication, Conflict, Leadership in an Interprofessional Team Environment

Integrating a New Team Member into a Community Healthcare Organization

Personnel

Judy: recently hired as a team social worker
Shirley: team RN
Fran: social work supervisor (administrative team)
Carol: team facilitator (administrative team)

Situation

Judy, who had worked as a senior social worker in a mental health setting for 12 years, was hired as a team social worker in a community healthcare organization. Shirley, one of the team RNs, perceived Judy as hesitant and ineffective in patient care-planning meetings. Other team members also found Judy to be too hesitant in making decisions, often rolling their eyes when Judy asked team members for their opinions. Despite their concerns about Judy's hesitancy, team members complained when Judy did not consult them before making patient-care decisions. As Judy experienced these mixed messages, she became more guarded in her social work assessments.

The IHT on which Judy was placed had a culture of socializing together after work. Initially, team members invited Judy to join them but Judy did not believe that socializing with colleagues was appropriate. In their socialization sessions the team discussed Judy's behavior, often noting that her mode of dress was out of style. Carol, a team facilitator, would occasionally join the rest of the team for a drink after work. Shirley complained to Carol that Judy was not doing her job. She also mentioned that the team did not like Judy, because she didn't socialize with them and wouldn't disclose information about her personal life as they all had done with each other. The nursing assistant and dietitian saw Judy as being very unfriendly. Subsequently, Carol spoke with Fran, stating that Judy was a problem and she wasn't sure that Judy would work out in the agency.

In her monthly supervisory meeting Fran asked Judy how things were going with her team. As Judy's eyes began to tear she said that she was thinking of leaving. Judy said that she was confident in her mental health experience, but not her team experience. She said that she hadn't realized how hard it would be to work with an IHT, and commented that the team members kept comparing her to a former team social worker who was not liked by the team. Judy told Fran that the team seemed uncomfortable with mental health issues and that she was shocked when the team made derogatory comments about patients (that some were dirty and smelly or that the team couldn't stand certain patients). In her conversation with Fran, Judy said the team had verbally chastised her for suggesting that a patient diagnosed by the internist as bipolar might not be bipolar. Judy was upset that she had expressed anger at the team while defending her assessment. Now Judy wasn't sure what to do because someone had told her that once you were on Shirley's bad side she would hate you forever.

Questions for Discussion

1. What are the central issues at stake in this case?
2. How do they affect the work of the IHT in deciding what to do in this situation?
3. How should these issues be resolved?
4. Is this solely a communication issue or is it a team development issue?
5. What kinds of leadership are needed in this case?
6. How should this situation be resolved?

Notes

Foreword

1. Okun, S., Schoenbaum, S., Andrews, D., Chidambaran, P., Chollette, V., Gruman, J., et al. (2014). *Patients and health care teams forging effective partnerships.* Discussion Paper, Institute of Medicine, Washington, D.C. Available at http://www.iom.edu/patientsaspartners. Accessed December 4, 2015.

2. Institute of Medicine. (1999). *To err is human: Building a safer health system.* Washington, DC: Author.

3. The Affordable Care Act. (2010). "Public Law 111–148." March 23, 2010. 111th U.S. Congress. Washington, DC: U.S. Government Printing Office.

4. Berwick, D. M., Nolan, T. W., and Whittington, J. (2008). The Triple Aim: Care, health, and cost. *Health Affairs, 27*: 759–769.

5. Okun et al., *Patients and health care teams.*

6. Interprofessional Education Collaborative. (2011). *Core competencies for interprofessional collaborative practice: Report of an expert panel.* Washington, DC: Author.

Foreword to the First Edition

1. Baldwin, D. C. (1996). Some historical notes on interdisciplinary and interprofessional education in practice in health care in the USA. *Journal of Interprofessional Care, 10*: 173–187.

Chapter 1

1. Available at http://www.webmd.com/children/vaccines/vaccines-what-todays-parents-should-know/vaccine-exemption-rates/default.htm. Accessed September 6, 2015.

2. Friedberg, M. W., Chen, P. G., White, C., Jung, O., Raaen, L., Hirshman, S., Hoch, E., Stevens, C., Ginsburg, P. B., Casalino, L. P., Tutty, M., Vargo, C., and Lipinski, L. (2015). Effects of health care payment models on physician practice in the United States. Rand Corporation, Santa Monica, CA.

3. Available at http://www.ihi.org/engage/initiatives/TripleAim/Pages/default .aspx. Accessed December 28, 2015.

4. Available at http://www.TeamSTEPPS.ahrq.gov. Accessed December 28, 2015.

5. Available at http://bhpr.hrsa.gov. Accessed March 4, 2016.

6. Available at http://www.macyfoundation.org. Accessed December 28, 2015.

7. Holmboe, E., Ginsburg, S., and Bernabeo, E. (2011). The rotational approach to medical education: Time to confront our assumptions. *Medical Education*, 45: 69–80.

Chapter 2

1. Mayes, R. (2007). The origins, development, and passage of Medicare's revolutionary prospective payment system. *Journal of the History of Medicine and Allied Sciences*, 62: 21–55.

2. Available at http://www.ncqa.org/Programs/Recognition/Practices/Patient CenteredMedicalHomePCMH.aspx. Accessed October 18, 2015.

3. TeamSTEPPS®. Agency for Healthcare Research and Quality, Rockville, MD. Available at http://www.ahrq.gov/cpi/about/otherwebsites/teamstepps/team stepps.html. Accessed September 20, 2015.

4. Grant, A. (2007). Relational job design and the motivation to make a prosocial difference. *Academy of Management Review*, 32 (2): 393–417.

5. Baccili, P. A. (2003). Effects of company and manager psychological contract violation on justice, negative affect and commitment. *Academy of Management Proceedings*, August 1: D1–D6. doi 10.5465/AMBPP.2003.13792579.

6. Tribble, S. J. (2015). Cleveland hospitals grapple with readmission fines. *Kaiser Health News*. WCPN, January 26. Available at http://www.khn.org. Accessed March 14, 2015.

Chapter 3

1. Elbing, A. O., Jr. (1970). The value issue of business: The responsibility of the businessman. *Academy of Management Journal*, 13: 79.

2. Steiner G. (1975). *Business and society*. New York: Random House.

3. Drinka, T. J. K., and Ray, R. O. (1992). Health care team ≠ Health care team. In J. R. Snyder (Ed.), *Proceedings of the fourteenth annual conference on interdisciplinary health care teams* (pp. 1–12). Indianapolis, IN: School of Allied Health Sciences, Indiana University Medical Center. Available at https://nexusipe .org. Accessed December 1, 2015.

4. Steffen, A. M., Zeiss, A. M., and Karel, M. J. (2014). Interprofessional geriatric healthcare: Competencies and resources for teamwork. In N. Pachana and K. Lardlaw (Eds.) *Oxford Handbook of clinical geropsychology: International perspectives* (pp. 733–752). Oxford: Oxford University Press.

5. Orsburn, J. D., Moran, L., Musselwhite, E., and Zenger, J. H. (1990). *Self-directed work teams: The new American challenge.* Homewood, IL: Business One Irwin.

6. TeamSTEPPS Curriculum. Available at http://www.ahrq.gov. Accessed September 15, 2015.

7. Charatan, F. B., Foley, C. J., and Libow, L. S. (1985). The team approach to geriatric medicine. In R. Andres, E. L. Bierman, and W. R. Hazzard (Eds.), *Principles of geriatric medicine* (pp. 169–175). New York: McGraw-Hill.

8. Drinka, T. J. K. (1996). Applying learning from self-directed work teams in business to curriculum development for interdisciplinary geriatric teams. *Educational Gerontology*, 22: 433–450.

9. Drinka, T. J. K. (1991). Development and maintenance of an interdisciplinary health care team: A case study. *Gerontology and Geriatrics Education*, 12: 111–127.

10. Lacoursiere, R. B. (1980). *The life cycle of groups: Group development stage theory.* New York: Human Sciences Press.

Chapter 4

1. Leonard, M., Graham, S., and Bonacum, D. (2004). The human factor: The critical importance of effective teamwork and communication in providing safe care. *Quality and Safety in Health,* 13: i85–i90.

2. *Houghton Mifflin Dictionary.* (2015). Available at www.dictionary.search.yahoo.com. Accessed December 1, 2015.

3. Schön, D. A. (1987). *Educating the reflective practitioner.* San Francisco, CA: Jossey-Bass.

4. Loftus, S., and Greenhalgh, T. (2010). Towards a narrative mode of practice. In J. Higgs, D. Fish, I. Goulter, S. Loftus, J.-A. Reid, and F. Trede (Eds.), *Education for future practice* (p. 86). Rotterdam, The Netherlands: Sense Publishers.

5. Almås, S. H., and Ødegård, A. (2010). Impact of professional cultures on students' perceptions of interprofessionalism. *Journal of Allied Health, 39*: 143–149.

6. Clark, P. G. (1995). Quality of life, values, and teamwork in geriatric care: Do we communicate what we mean? *The Gerontologist, 35*: 402–411.

7. Clark, P. G. (1997). Values in health care professional socialization: Implications for geriatric education in interdisciplinary teamwork. *The Gerontologist, 37*: 441–451.

8. Sims, D. (2011). Reconstructing professional identity for professional and interprofessional practice: A mixed methods study of joint training programmes

in learning disability nursing and social work. *Journal of Interprofessional Care*, *25*: 265–271.

9. Clandinin, D. J., and Cave, M.-T. (2008). Creating pedagogical spaces for developing doctor professional identity. *Medical Education*, *42*: 765–770.

10. Poirier, S. (2002). Voice in the medical narrative. In R. Charon and M. Montello (Eds.), *Stories matter: The role of narrative in medical ethics* (pp. 48–58). New York: Routledge.

11. Walker, M. (2007). *Moral understandings* (2nd ed.). New York: Oxford University Press.

12. Lingard, L., Schryer, C. F., Spafford, M. M., and Campbell, S. L. (2007). Negotiating the politics of identity in an interdisciplinary research team. *Qualitative Research*, *7*: 501–519.

13. Loftus and Greenhalgh, Towards a narrative mode of practice, p. 90.

14. Goldsmith, J., Wittenberg-Lyles, E., Rodriguez, D., and Sanchez-Reilly, S. (2010). Interdisciplinary geriatric and palliative care team narratives: Collaboration practices and barriers. *Qualitative Health Research*, *20*: 93–104.

15. Haidet, P., and Paterniti, D. A. (2003). "Building" a history rather than "taking" one: A perspective on information sharing during the medical interview. *Archives of Internal Medicine*, *163:* 1134–1140.

16. Waitzkin, H., Britt, T., and Williams, C. (1994). Narratives of aging and social problems in medical encounters with older persons. *Journal of Health and Social Behavior*, *35:* 340.

17. Graybeal, C. (2001). Strengths-based social work assessment: Transforming the dominant paradigm. *Families in Society: The Journal of Contemporary Human Services*, *82*: 233–242.

18. Qualls, S. H., and Czirr, R. (1988). Geriatric health teams: Classifying models of professional and team functioning. *The Gerontologist*, *28*: 372–376.

19. Hebert, C. P. (2005). Changing the culture: Interprofessional education for collaborative patient-centred practice in Canada. *Journal of Interprofessional Care*, *19* (Suppl. 1): 1–4.

20. Clarke, A. (2000). Using biography to enhance the nursing care of older people. *British Journal of Nursing*, *9*: 698.

21. Qualls and Czirr, Geriatric health teams.

22. Lingard et al., Negotiating the politics of identity.

23. Walker, *Moral understandings*.

24. Gaydos, H. L. (2005). Understanding personal narratives: An approach to practice. *Journal of Advanced Nursing*, *49*: 255.

25. Graybeal, Strengths-based social work assessment.

26. Nelson, H. L. (1999). Stories of my old age. In M. Walker (Ed.), *Mother time: Women, aging, and ethics* (p. 85). New York: Rowman & Littlefield.

27. Hsu, M. Y., and McCormack, B. (2011). Using narrative inquiry with older people to inform practice and service developments. *Journal of Clinical Nursing*, *21:* 841–849.

28. Poirier, Voice in the medical narrative.

29. Holstein, M. B., Parks, J. A., and Waymack, M. H. (2011). *Ethics, aging, and society: The critical turn* (p. 41). New York: Springer.

30. Hazelton, L. (2010). "I check my emotions the way you might check a pulse . . .": Stories of women doctors. *Storytelling, Self, Society, 6*: 132–144.

31. McClelland, M., and Sands, R. G. (1993). The missing voice in interdisciplinary communication. *Qualitative Health Research, 3*: 74–90.

32. Opie, A. (1997). Thinking teams thinking clients: Issues of discourse and representation in the work of health care teams. *Sociology of Health & Illness, 19*: 259–280.

33. Dickey, L. A., Truten, J., Gross, L. M., and Deitrick, L. M. (2011). Promotion of staff resiliency and interdisciplinary team cohesion through two small-group narrative exchange models designed to facilitate patient- and family-centered care. *Journal of Communication in Health Care, 4*: 126–138.

34. Sands, S. A., Stanley, P., and Charon, R. (2008). Pediatric narrative oncology: Interprofessional training to promote empathy, build teams, and prevent burnout. *Journal of Supportive Oncology, 6:* 307–312.

35. Blickem, C., and Priyadharshini, E. (2007). Patient narratives: The potential for "patient-centred" interprofessional learning? *Journal of Interprofessional Care, 21*: 619–632.

36. Medical jargon. Available at http://www.ruf.rice.edu/~kemmer/words04/usage/jargon_medical.html. Accessed September 28, 2015.

37. Top 47 slang terms nurses use. (2011). *Scrubs: The Nurses Guide to Good Living, July, 8.* Available at http://www.scrubsmag.com/. Accessed September 28, 2015.

38. Nursing acronyms and abbreviations: 993 acronyms and abbreviations related to nursing. Available at http://www.allacronyms.com/. Accessed September 28, 2015.

39. Moseley, V. (2014). Social workers: Watch your language. *Social Work Helper. September 2.* Available at http://www.socialworkhelper.com/. Accessed September 28, 2015.

40. Columbia University School of Social Work. Human Service Acronyms. Available at http://www.socialwork.columbia.edu/. Accessed September 28, 2015.

41. The MBA jargon index. MBA Jargon Watch. Available at http://www.johnsmurf.com/. Accessed September 28, 2015.

42. Ryan, L. (2014). What business jargon says about us, Forbes.com, October 1. Available at http://www.forbes.com/sites/lizryan/2014/10/1what-business-jargon-says-about-us/. Accessed September 28, 2015.

43. TeamSTEPPS 2.0 Course Management Guide, Agency for Healthcare Research and Quality. Available at http://www.ahrq.gov/. Accessed September 28, 2015.

44. Lakoff, G., and Johnson, M. (1980). *Metaphors we live by.* Chicago, IL: University of Chicago Press.

45. Drinka, T. J. K., and Miller, T. F. (1996). The health care team as metaphor: A preliminary study. *Journal of Allied Health, 25* (3): 247–261.

Chapter 5

1. Drinka, T. J. K. (1991). *A case study of leadership on a long term interdisciplinary health care team.* (Doctoral dissertation, University of Wisconsin, Madison, 1990). *Dissertation Abstracts International, 51*: 11, 3599A.

2. Romig, D. A. (1996). *Breakthrough teamwork.* Chicago, IL: Irwin.

3. Drinka, T., and Ray, R. O. (1986). An investigation of power in an interdisciplinary health care team. *Gerontology & Geriatrics Education, 6* (3): 43–53.

4. Kaluzny, A. (1985). Design and management of disciplinary and interdisciplinary groups in health services: Review and critique. *Medical Care Review, 42*: 77–112.

5. Anderson, O., and Gevitz, N. (1983). The general hospital: A social and historical perspective. In D. Mechanic (Ed.), *Handbook of health, health care, and the health professions* (pp. 305–317). New York: Free Press.

6. Drinka, *A case study of leadership.*

7. Drinka, T. J. K., and Goodman, B. M. (2002). Perceptions of self and team development among members of interdisciplinary teams in health and human services. Presented at the Combined Interdisciplinary Healthcare Team and National Academies of Practice Conference, April 12–13, Arlington, VA.

8. Rittel, H., and Webber, M. (1973). Dilemmas in a general theory of planning. *Policy Sciences, 4*: 155–169.

9. Cannon-Bowers, J. A., and Salas, E. (2001). Reflections on shared cognition. *Journal of Organizational Behavior, 22*: 195–202.

10. Marks, M. A., Sabella, M. J., Burke, C. S., and Zacarro, S. J. (2002). The impact of cross-training on team effectiveness. *Journal of Applied Psychology, 87*: 3–13.

11. Healey, M. P., Vuori, T., and Hodgkinson, G. P. (2015). When teams agree while disagreeing: Reflexion and reflection in shared cognition. *Academy of Management Review, 40*: 399–422.

12. Hackman, J. R. (1998). Why teams don't work. In R. S. Tinsdale, J. Edwards, and E. J. Posavac (Eds.), *Theory and research on small groups* (pp. 245–267). New York: Plenum.

Chapter 6

1. Bolman, L. G., and Deal, T. E. (2013). *Modern approaches to understanding and managing organizations* (5th ed.). San Francisco, CA: Jossey-Bass.

2. Morgan, G. (1997). *Images of organization* (2nd ed.). Thousand Oaks, CA: Sage.

3. Bass, B. M., and Bass, R. (2008). *The Bass handbook of leadership: Theory, research, and managerial applications* (4th ed.). New York: Free Press.

4. Bennis, W. G. (1965). Theory and method in applying behavioral science to planned organizational change. *Journal of Applied Behavioral Science, 1*: 337–360.

NOTES   295

5. Morgan, *Images of organization.*

6. Baldwin, D. C. (1996). Some historical notes on interdisciplinary and interprofessional education and practice in health care in the USA. *Journal of Interprofessional Care, 10*: 173–187.

7. Katz, D., and Kahn, R. L. (1978). *The social psychology of organizations* (2nd ed., pp. 527–528). New York: Wiley and Sons.

8. Pfeffer, J. (1981). *Power in organizations.* Marshfield, MA: Pitman Publishing.

9. Drinka, T. J. K. (1987). Interdisciplinary health team and organizational development literature: An analysis of approaches to conflict recognition, resolution, and management. In M. L. Brunner and R. M. Casto (Eds.), *Interdisciplinary health team care: Proceedings of the eighth annual conference* (pp. 74–84). Columbus, OH: School of Allied Medical Professions and Commission on Interprofessional Education and Practice, The Ohio State University. Available at https://nexusipe.org. Accessed March 17, 2016.

10. Bolman and Deal, *Modern approaches.*

11. Drinka, T. J. K. (1986). Unpublished data.

12. Drinka, T. J. K, and Miller, T. F. (1996). The health care team as metaphor: A preliminary study. *Journal of Allied Health, 25* (3): 245–261.

13. Katz and Kahn, *The social psychology of organizations.*

14. Cartwright, D., and Zander, A. (1968). *Group dynamics: Research and method* (3rd ed.). New York: Harper and Row.

15. Vroom, V. H., and Jago, A. G. (1988). *The new leadership: Managing participation in organizations.* Englewood Cliffs, NJ: Prentice-Hall.

16. Schön, D. A. (1984). Leadership as reflection in action. In T. J. Sergiovanni and J. E. Corbally (Eds.), *Leadership and organizational culture: New perspectives on administrative theory and practice* (pp. 36–63). Chicago: University of Illinois Press.

17. Terman, L. M. (1904). A preliminary study of the psychology and pedagogy of leadership. *Journal of Genetic Psychology, 11*: 413–451.

18. Stogdill, R. M. (1948). Personal factors associated with leadership: A survey of the literature. *Journal of Psychology, 25*: 35–71.

19. Lewin, K. R., Lippitt, R., and White, R. K. (1939). Patterns of aggressive behavior in experimentally created social climates. *Journal of Social Psychology, 10*: 271–299.

20. Stogdill, R. M., and A. E. Coons (Eds.) (1957). *Leader behavior: Its description and measurement.* Columbus, OH: Bureau of Business Research, The Ohio State University.

21. Yukl, G. A., and Nemeroff, W. (1979). Identification and measurement of specific categories of leadership behavior: A progress report. In J. G. Hunt and L. L. Larson (Eds.). *Crosscurrents in leadership.* Carbondale, IL: Southern Illinois State University Press.

22. Bales, R. F., and Slater, P. (1955). Role differentiation in small social groups. In T. Parsons, R. F. Bales, and E. A. Shils (Eds.), *Family, socialization and interaction process* (pp. 259–306). Glencoe, IL: Free Press.

23. Hersey, P., and Blanchard, K. (1982). *Management of organizational behavior: Utilizing human resources* (4th ed). Englewood Cliffs, NJ: Prentice-Hall.

24. Hollander, E. P. (1964). *Leaders, groups, and influence.* New York: Oxford University Press.

25. House, R. J. (1971). A path-goal theory of leader effectiveness. *Administrative Science Quarterly, 16*: 321–338.

26. Graen, G., Novak, M. A., and Sommerkamp, P. (1982). The effects of leader-member exchange and job design on productivity and satisfaction: Testing a dual attachment model. *Organizational Behavior and Human Performance, 30*: 109–131.

27. Hollander, E. P. (1979). Leadership and social exchange processes. In K. J. Gergen, M. S. Greenberg, and R. H. Willis (Eds.). *Social exchange: Advances in theory and research* (pp. 103–118). New York: Winston-Wiley.

28. Bass, B. M. (1990). *Bass and Stogdill's handbook of leadership: Theory, research and managerial applications* (3rd ed.). New York: Free Press.

29. Smith, P. B., and Peterson, M. F. (1988). *Leadership, organizations, and culture.* London: Sage.

30. Calder, B. J. (1977). An attribution theory of leadership. In B. M. Staw and G. R. Salancik (Eds.), *New directions in organizational behavior* (pp. 179–204). Chicago, IL: St. Clair Press.

31. Smith and Peterson, *Leadership, organizations.*

32. Argyris, C. (1982). *Reasoning, learning, and action: Individual and organizational.* San Francisco, CA: Jossey-Bass.

33. Argyris, C., Putnam, R., and Smith, D. M. (1987). *Action science.* San Francisco, CA: Jossey-Bass.

34. Foti, R. J., Fraser, S. L., and Lord, R. G. (1982). Effects of leadership labels and prototypes on perceptions of political leaders. *Journal of Applied Psychology, 67*: 326–333.

35. Bass, B. M., Waldman, D. A., Avolio, B. J., and Bebb, M. (1987). Transformational leadership and the falling dominoes effect. *Group and Organization Studies, 12:* 73–87.

36. Bennis, W., and Nanus, B. (1985). *Leaders: The strategies for taking charge.* New York: Harper and Row.

37. Burns, J. M. (1978). *Leadership.* New York: Harper and Row.

38. Smith and Peterson, *Leadership, organizations.*

39. Raelin, J. (2006). Does action learning promote collaborative leadership? *Academy of Management Learning and Education, 5* (2): 152–168.

40. Hollander, E. P. (1961). Some effects of perceived status on responses to innovative behavior. *Journal of Abnormal and Social Psychology, 63*: 247–250.

41. Fisher, B. A. (1986). Leadership: When does the difference make a difference? In R. A. Hirakawa and M. S. Poole (Eds.), *Communication and group decision-making* (pp. 197–215). Beverly Hills: Sage.

42. Jago, A. G. (1982). Perspectives in theory and research. *Management Science, 28*: 315–336.

43. Ibid., p. 315.

44. Schön, Leadership as reflection in action.

45. Morgan, *Images of organization.*

46. Vroom, V. H., and Jago, A. G. (1988). *The new leadership: Managing participation in organizations.* Englewood Cliffs, NJ: Prentice-Hall.

47. Lombardo, M. M. (1978). *Looking at leadership: Some neglected issues* (Technical Report Number 6). Greensboro, NC: Center for Creative Leadership.

48. Salancik, G. J., and Pfeffer, J. (1977). Who gets power—and how they hold on to it: A strategic contingency model of power. *Organizational Dynamics,* 5: 3–21.

49. Parsons, T. (1960). *Structure and process in modern societies.* New York: Free Press.

50. Drinka, T., and Ray, R. O. (1986). An investigation of power in an interdisciplinary health care team. *Gerontology & Geriatrics Education, 6* (3): 43–53.

51. Drinka, T. J. K. (1991). A case study of leadership on a long term interdisciplinary health care team. (Doctoral dissertation, University of Wisconsin–Madison, 1990). *Dissertation Abstracts International, 51* (11): 3599A.

52. Hickson, G. B., Pichert, J. W., Webb, L. E., and Gabbe, S. G, (2007). A complementary approach to promoting professionalism: Identifying, measuring, and addressing unprofessional behaviors. *Academic Medicine, 82*: 1040–1048.

53. Drinka, A case study of leadership.

54. Drinka, T. J. K., and Miller, T. F. (1996). The health care team as metaphor: A preliminary study. *Journal of Allied Health, 25* (3): 247–261.

55. Drinka, A case study of leadership.

56. Ibid.

57. Beckhouse, L. S., Tanur, J., Weiler, J., and Weinstein, E. (1975). And some men have leadership thrust upon them. *Journal of Personality and Social Psychology, 31*: 557–566.

58. Drinka, A case study of leadership.

Chapter 7

1. Boulding, K. (1963). *Conflict and defense.* New York: Harper and Row.

2. Blake, R. R., and Mouton, J. S. (1984). *Solving costly organizational conflicts.* San Francisco, CA: Jossey-Bass.

3. Smith, K. K., and Berg, D. N. (1987). *Paradoxes of group life.* San Francisco, CA: Jossey-Bass.

4. Janss, R., Rispens, S., Segers, M., and Jehn, K. A. (2012). Power, conflict and the performance of medical teams. *Medical Education, 46*: 838–849.

5. Grer, L. L., Saygi, O., Aaldering, H., and de Dreu, C. K. W. (2012). Conflict in medical teams: Opportunity or danger? *Medical Education, 46*: 935–942.

6. Jehn, K. A., and Mannix, E. A. (2001). The dynamic nature of conflict: A longitudinal study of intragroup conflict and group performance. *Academy of Management Journal, 44*: 238–251.

7. Kane, R. A. (1975). *Interprofessional teamwork* (Manpower Monograph No. 8). Syracuse, NY: Division of Continuing Education and Manpower Development of the Syracuse University School of Social Work.

8. Brown, J., Lewis, L., Ellis, K., Stewart, M., and Freeman, T. R. (2011). Conflict on interprofessional primary health care teams—Can it be resolved? *Journal of Interprofessional Care*, 25: 4–10.

9. Grer, Saygi, Aaldering, and de Dreu, Conflict in medical teams.

10. Drinka, T. J. K. (1987). Interdisciplinary health team and organizational development literature: An analysis of approaches to conflict recognition, resolution, and management. In M. L. Brunner and R. M. Casto (Eds.), *Interdisciplinary health team care: Proceedings of the eighth annual conference* (pp. 74–84). Columbus, OH: School of Allied Medical Professions and Commission on Interprofessional Education and Practice, The Ohio State University. Available through https://nexusipe.org. Accessed December 15, 2015.

11. Drinka, T. J. K. (1994). Interdisciplinary geriatric teams: Approaches to conflict as indicators of potential to model teamwork. *Educational Gerontology*, 20: 87–103.

12. Ibid.

13. Mayer, R. C., Davis, J. H., and Schoorman, F. D. (1995). An integrative model of organizational trust. *Academy of Management Review*, 20: 709–734.

14. Bachmann, R., and Zaheer, A. (Eds.). (2006). *Handbook of trust research*. Cheltenham, UK: Edward Elgar.

15. Simons, T. L. (2002). Behavioral integrity—The perceived alignment between managers' words and deeds as a research focus. *Organization Science*, 13: 18–35.

16. Drinka, T. J. K., and Goodman, B. M. (2004). The team signatures technology: A conceptual framework. Presented at the All Together Better Health Conference, Vancouver, BC, Canada, May 7, 2004.

17. Ring, P. S., and Van de Ven, A. H. (1994). Developmental processes of cooperative interorganizational relationships. *Academy of Management Review*, 19: 90–118.

18. Drinka, T. J. K., Miller, T., and Goodman, B. M. (1996). Characterizing motivational styles of professionals who work on interdisciplinary healthcare teams. *Journal of Interprofessional Care*, 10: 51–61.

19. Blake, R. R., and Mouton, J. S. (1964). *The managerial grid*. Houston: Gulf.

20. Thomas, K. W. (1977). Toward multi-dimensional values in teaching: The example of conflict behaviors. *Academy of Management Review*, 12: 484–490.

21. Grer, Saygi, Aaldering, and de Dreu, Conflict in medical teams.

22. Drinka, T. J. K. (1991). A case study of leadership on a long term interdisciplinary health care team. (Doctoral dissertation, University of Wisconsin–Madison, 1990). *Dissertation Abstracts International*, 51 (11): 3599A.

23. Hall, J. (1986). *Conflict management survey*. Woodlands, TX: Teleometrics International.

24. Drinka, A case study of leadership on a long term interdisciplinary health care team.

25. Federation of State Medical Boards of the United States, Inc. (2000). Report of the Special Committee on Professional Conduct and Ethics. Dallas, TX: Federation of State Medical Boards.

26. Leape, L. L., and Fromson, J. A. (2006). Problem doctors: Is there a system-level solution? *Annals of Internal Medicine, 144*: 107–115.

27. Rosenstein, A. H., and O'Daniel, M. (2005). Disruptive behavior and clinical outcomes. *American Journal of Nursing, 105* (1): 54–64.

28. Drinka, T. J. K., and Streim, J. E. (1994). Case studies from purgatory: Maladaptive behavior within geriatrics health care teams, *The Gerontologist, 34*: 541–547.

29. Drinka, T. J. K., and Synnes, J. (2011). *Stung by "B"s: A storybook on how to recognize and survive venomous behaviors.* Waupaca, WI: Bbalm Publishing.

30. Drinka and Streim, Case studies from purgatory.

31. Drinka and Synnes, *Stung by "B"s.*

32. Morgan, G. (1989). *Creative organization theory.* Thousand Oaks, CA: Sage.

33. Drinka, A case study of leadership on a long-term interdisciplinary health care team.

Chapter 8

1. Hibbard, J. H., and Greene, J. (2013). What the evidence shows about patient activation: Better health outcomes and care experiences; fewer data on costs. *Health Affairs, 32*: 207–214.

2. Veroff, D., Marr, A., and Wennberg, D. E. (2013). Enhanced support for shared decision making reduced costs of care for patient with preference-sensitive conditions. *Health Affairs, 32* (2): 285–293.

3. Clayton, E. W. (2003). Ethical, legal, and social implication of genomics. *New England Journal of Medicine, 349*: 562–569.

4. Available at http://www.ahrq.gov/patients-consumers/index.html. Accessed December 15, 2015

5. Robbins, A. (2015). *The nurses: A year of secrets, drama, and miracles with the heroes of the hospital.* New York: Workman Publishing.

6. Arts, D. G. T., de Keizer, N. F., and Scheffer, G.-J. (2002). Defining and improving data quality in medical registries: A literature review, case study, and generic framework. *Journal of the American Medical Informatics Association, 9*: 600–611.

7. Terry, K. J., and Fiore, M. (September 22, 2014). Doctors willing to share medical practice with patients? Sort of. *Medscape Business of Medicine.* Available at http://www.medscape.com. Accessed November 25, 2015

8. Reeve, J. (2010). Interpretive medicine: Supporting generalism in a changing primary care world. *Occasional Paper (Royal College of General Practitioners), 88*: 1–20.

9. Howell, T. (2015). The Wisconsin Star Method: Understanding and addressing complexity in geriatrics. In Malone, M. L., Capezuti, E., and Palmer, R. M. (Eds.), *Geriatric models of care: Bringing 'best practice' to an aging America* (pp. 87–94). Cham, Switzerland: Springer International Publishing.

Chapter 9

1. Institute of Medicine. (2012). *Core principles and values of effective team-based health care*. Washington, DC: Author.

2. Interprofessional Education Collaborative. (2011). *Core competencies for interprofessional collaborative practice: Report of an expert panel*. Washington, DC: Author.

3. Qualls, S. H., and Czirr, R. (1988). Geriatric health teams: Classifying models of professional and team functioning. *The Gerontologist, 28*: 372–376.

4. Gadow, S. (1983). Frailty and strength: The dialectic in aging. *The Gerontologist, 23*: 144–147.

5. Kayser-Jones, J. S. (1986). Distributive justice and the treatment of acute illness in nursing homes. *Social Science and Medicine, 23*: 1279–1286.

6. Gramelspacher, G. P., Howell, J. D., and Young, M. J. (1986). Perceptions of ethical problems by nurses and doctors. *Archives of Internal Medicine, 146*: 577–578.

7. Walker, R. M., Miles, S. H., Stocking, C. B., and Siegler, M. (1991). Physicians' and nurses' perceptions of ethics problems on general medical services. *Journal of General Internal Medicine, 6*: 424–429.

8. Jones, J. M., Meredith, S., Wadas, L., Watt, S., and Weisz, E. (1991). The contribution and role of the social worker. In National Advisory Council on Aging (Ed.), *Geriatric assessment and treatment: Members of the team* (pp. 35–52). No. H71-2/1-9-1991E. Ottawa, ON: Minister of Supply and Services Canada.

9. Institute of Medicine, *Core principles and values*.

10. Winkler, E. C., and Gruen, R. L. (2005). First principles: Substantive ethics for healthcare organizations. *Journal of Healthcare Management, 50*: 109–119.

11. Melia, K. M. (2001). Ethical issues and the importance of consensus for the intensive care team. *Social Science and Medicine, 53*: 707–719.

12. Moody, H. R. (1988). From informed consent to negotiated consent. *The Gerontologist, 28* (Suppl.): 64–70.

13. Thomasma, D. (1982). Moral education in interdisciplinary teams. *Surgical Technologies, 2*: 17. Cited in Purtilo, R. B. (1988). Ethical issues in teamwork: The context of rehabilitation. *Archives of Physical Medicine and Rehabilitation, 69*: 321.

Chapter 10

1. Lewin, K. (1951). *Field theory in social science: Selected theoretical papers* (D. Cartwright, Ed (p. 169). New York: Harper and Row.

2. Baldwin, D. C. (2000). Foreword. In T. J. K. Drinka and P. G. Clark, *Health care teamwork: Interdisciplinary practice and teaching* (p. xii). Westport, CT: Auburn House/Greenwood.

3. Proust, M. (1981). The captive. In C. K. Moncrieff, R. Kilmartin, and A. Mayor (Trans.), *Remembrance of things past* (Vol. 3, p. 260). New York: Random House.

4. Institute of Medicine. (2015). *Measuring the impact of interprofessional education on collaborative practice and patient outcomes.* Washington, DC: Author.

5. Bengtson, V. L., Rice, C. J., and Johnson, M. L. (1999). Are theories of aging important? Models and explanations in gerontology at the turn of the century. In V. L. Bengtson and K. W. Schaie (Eds.), *Handbook of theories of aging* (p. 5). New York: Springer.

6. Barr, H., Koppel, I., Reeves, S., Hammick, M., and Freeth, D. (2005). *Effective interprofessional education: Argument, assumption, and evidence* (p. 120). Oxford, UK: Blackwell.

7. Barr et al., *Effective interprofessional education*, p. 31.

8. Dahlgren, L. O. (2006, April). Developing flexibility through experiencing variety: A potential function of interprofessional learning for improving competence. Paper presented at the All Together Better Health III Conference: Challenges in Education and Practice, London, UK.

9. Kolb, D. A. (1984). *Experiential learning.* Englewood Cliffs, NJ: Prentice-Hall.

10. Petrie, H. G. (1976). Do you see what I see? The epistemology of interdisciplinary inquiry. *Journal of Aesthetic Education, 10*: 29–43.

11. Clark, P. G. (1995). Quality of life, values, and teamwork in geriatric care: Do we communicate what we mean? *The Gerontologist, 35*: 402–411.

12. Clark, P. G. (1997). Values in health care professional socialization: Implications for geriatric education in interdisciplinary teamwork. *The Gerontologist, 37*: 441–451.

13. Becher, T. (1989). *Academic tribes and territories: Intellectual enquiry and the cultures of disciplines.* Bristol, PA: The Society for Research into Higher Education and Open University Press.

14. Lattuca, L. R. (2002). Learning interdisciplinarity: Sociocultural perspectives on academic work. *Journal of Higher Education, 73*: 711–739.

15. Dahlgren, Developing flexibility through experiencing variety.

16. Kolb, *Experiential learning.*

17. Clark, P. G. (2009). Reflecting on reflection in interprofessional education: Implications for theory and practice. *Journal of Interprofessional Care, 23*: 213–223.

18. Wackerhausen, S. (2006, September). Collaboration and reflection across boundaries. Paper presented at the Nordic Conference on Interprofessional Education and Collaboration, Breaking Boundaries—Building Bridges, Holstebro, Denmark.

19. Kolb, *Experiential learning*.

20. Schön, D. A. (1987). *Educating the reflective practitioner*. San Francisco, CA: Jossey-Bass.

21. Clark, P. G. (1994). Learning on interdisciplinary gerontological teams: Instructional concepts and methods. *Educational Gerontology, 20*: 349–364.

22. Clark, Reflecting on reflection.

23. Chan, W.-T. (1963). *The way of Lao Tzu* (p. 159). Indianapolis, IN: Bobbs-Merrill.

24. Clark, Reflecting on reflection.

Chapter 11

1. Satin, D. G. (1987). The difficulties of interdisciplinary education: Lessons from three failures and a success. *Educational Gerontology, 13*: 66.

2. Baldwin, D. C. (1996). Some historical notes on interdisciplinary and interprofessional education and practice in health care in the USA. *Journal of Interprofessional Care, 10*: 182.

3. Institute of Medicine. (2000). *To err is human: Building a safer health system*. Washington, DC: Author.

4. Institute of Medicine. (2001). *Crossing the quality chasm: A new health system for the 21st century*. Washington, DC: Author.

5. Institute of Medicine. (2003). *Health professions education: A bridge to quality*. Washington, DC: Author.

6. Institute of Medicine. (2015). *Measuring the impact of interprofessional education on collaborative practice and patient outcomes*. Washington, DC: Author.

7. Interprofessional Education Collaborative. (2011). *Core competencies for interprofessional collaborative practice: Report of an expert panel*. Washington, DC: Author.

8. Institute of Medicine. (2008). *Retooling for an aging society*. Washington, DC: Author.

9. Partnership for Health in Aging. (2014). Position statement on interdisciplinary team training in geriatrics: An essential component of quality health care for older adults. *Journal of the American Geriatrics Society, 62*: 961–965.

10. Patient-Centered Primary Care Collaborative. (2014). Progress and promise: Profiles in interprofessional health training to deliver patient-centered primary care. Available at www.pcpcc.org. Accessed on February 29, 2016.

11. Lattuca, L. R. (2002). Learning interdisciplinarity: Sociocultural perspectives on academic work. *Journal of Higher Education, 73*: 711–739.

12. Nikitina, S. (2005). Pathways of interdisciplinary cognition. *Cognition and Instruction, 23*: 389–425.

13. Klein, J. T. (1990). *Interdisciplinarity: History, theory, and practice.* Detroit, MI: Wayne State University Press.

14. Weingart, P., and Stehr, N. (2000). *Practising interdisciplinarity.* Toronto: University of Toronto Press.

15. Satin, The difficulties of interdisciplinary education, p. 65.

16. Abbott, A. (1988). *The system of professions: An essay on the division of expert labor.* Chicago, IL: University of Chicago Press.

17. Freidson, E. (1986). *Professional powers: A study of the institutionalization of formal knowledge.* Chicago, IL: University of Chicago Press.

18. Reuben, D. B., Levy-Storms, L., Yee, M. N., Lee, M., Cole, K., Waite, M., et al. (2004). Disciplinary split: A threat to geriatrics interdisciplinary team training. *Journal of the American Geriatrics Society, 52:* 1000–1006.

19. Gardner, S. F., Chamberlin, G. D., Heestand, D. E., and Stowe, C. D. (2002). Interdisciplinary didactic instruction at Academic Health Centers in the United States: Attitudes and barriers. *Advances in Health Sciences Education, 7:* 179–190.

20. Leipzig, R. M., Hyer, K., Ek, K., Wallenstein, S., Vezina, M. L., Fairchild, S., et al. (2002). Attitudes toward working on interdisciplinary healthcare teams: A comparison by discipline. *Journal of the American Geriatrics Society, 50:* 1141–1148.

21. Reuben et al., Disciplinary split.

22. Baker, L., Egan-Lee, E., Martimianakis, M. A., and Reeves, S. (2011). Relationships of power: Implications for interprofessional education. *Journal of Interprofessional Care, 25:* 98–104.

23. Satin, The difficulties of interdisciplinary education.

24. Barr, J., and Ross, F. (2006). Mainstreaming interprofessional education in the United Kingdom: A position paper. *Journal of Interprofessional Care, 20:* 103.

25. Lewin, K. (1951). *Field theory in social science.* New York: Harper and Row.

26. Prochaska J. O., and Velicer W. F. (1997). The transtheoretical model of health behavior change. *American Journal of Health Promotion, 12:* 38–48.

27. Prochaska, J. M. (2000). A transtheoretical model for assessing organizational change. *Families in Society, 81:* 76–84.

28. Prochaska, J. M., Prochaska, J. O., and Levesque, D. A. (2001). A transtheoretical approach to changing organizations. *Administration and Policy in Mental Health, 28:* 247–261.

29. Kezar, A., and Lester, J. (2009). *Organizing higher education for collaboration.* San Francisco, CA: Jossey-Bass.

30. Kezar, A., and Elrod, S. (2012). Facilitating interdisciplinary learning. *Change: The Magazine of Higher Learning* (pp. 16–25), January/February.

31. Ginsburg, L., and Tregunno, D. (2005). New approaches to interprofessional education and collaborative practice: Lessons from the organizational change literature. *Journal of Interprofessional Care, 19* (Suppl. 1): 177–187.

32. Hanson, M. (2001). Institutional theory and educational change. *Educational Administration Quarterly*, *37*: 637–661.

33. Caruso, D., and Rhoten, D. (2001). *Lead, follow, get out of the way: Sidestepping the barriers to effective practice of interdisciplinarity*. Hybrid Institute White Paper. Available at www.hybridvigor.org. Accessed on December 1, 2015.

34. Kezar and Elrod, Facilitating interdisciplinary learning.

35. DiMaggio, P. J., and Powell, W. W. (1983). The iron cage revisited: Institutional isomorphism and collective rationality in organization fields. *American Sociological Review*, *48*: 147–160.

36. Ginsburg and Tregunno, New approaches to interprofessional education.

37. Institute of Medicine, *Measuring the impact of interprofessional education.*

38. Ibid.

39. Satin, The difficulties of interdisciplinary education, p. 67.

Chapter 12

1. Frenk, J., Chen, L., Bhutta, Z. A., Cohen, J., Crisp, N., Evans, T., et al. (2010). Health professionals for a new century. *The Lancet, 376*: 1923–1958.

2. Institute of Medicine. (2015). *Measuring the impact of interprofessional education on collaborative practice and patient outcomes*. Washington, DC: Author.

Index

About the Authors

Theresa J. K. Drinka, PhD, MSSW, LCSW, is President of Drinka Consulting and Training, a consulting and training business for human systems analysis and team development in healthcare systems. She formerly was Director of Interprofessional Team Training and Associate Director and Co-Founder of the Geriatric Research Education and Clinical Center at the William S. Middleton Memorial Veterans Hospital, Madison, Wisconsin, developing and administering interprofessional clinical and education programs and performing clinical social work and research at the University of Wisconsin and the Department of Veterans Affairs. Dr. Drinka was instrumental in developing clinical assessment, training, and team evaluation methodologies including the *Team Signatures®*, a technology to help consultants evaluate the system dynamics of teams. She is coauthor of the award-winning *Stung by "B"s: A Storybook on How to Recognize and Survive Venomous Behaviors* and articles and book chapters on self-directed work teams, mental health, interprofessional healthcare teams, and patient assessment instruments.

Phillip G. Clark, ScD, is Professor and Director of both the Program in Gerontology and the Rhode Island Geriatric Education Center at the University of Rhode Island, where he has been on the faculty since 1981. He was awarded a Doctorate in Public Health from Harvard University in 1979, and during 1980–1981 was a Post-Doctoral Fellow in Ethics and Public Policy at Wesleyan University. He has served as a Visiting Professor at the Universities of Guelph and Toronto in Canada (1988–1989), a Fulbright Scholar at Buskerud University College in Norway (2007), and a Visiting Professor at the University of Huddersfield and Bournemouth University in England (2013). His experience includes teaching healthcare teamwork, developing interprofessional healthcare research and demonstration projects, and consulting on interprofessional educational development and evaluation in the United States, Canada, and Europe. His work has been published in *The Gerontologist, Canadian Journal on Aging, Journal of Aging Studies, Ageing and Society, Educational Gerontology, Gerontology and Geriatrics Education*, and the *Journal of Interprofessional Care*. Clark has served as Principal Investigator or Co-Investigator on over $17 million in grants, and he is a Fellow of both the Gerontological Society of America and the Association for Gerontology in Higher Education.